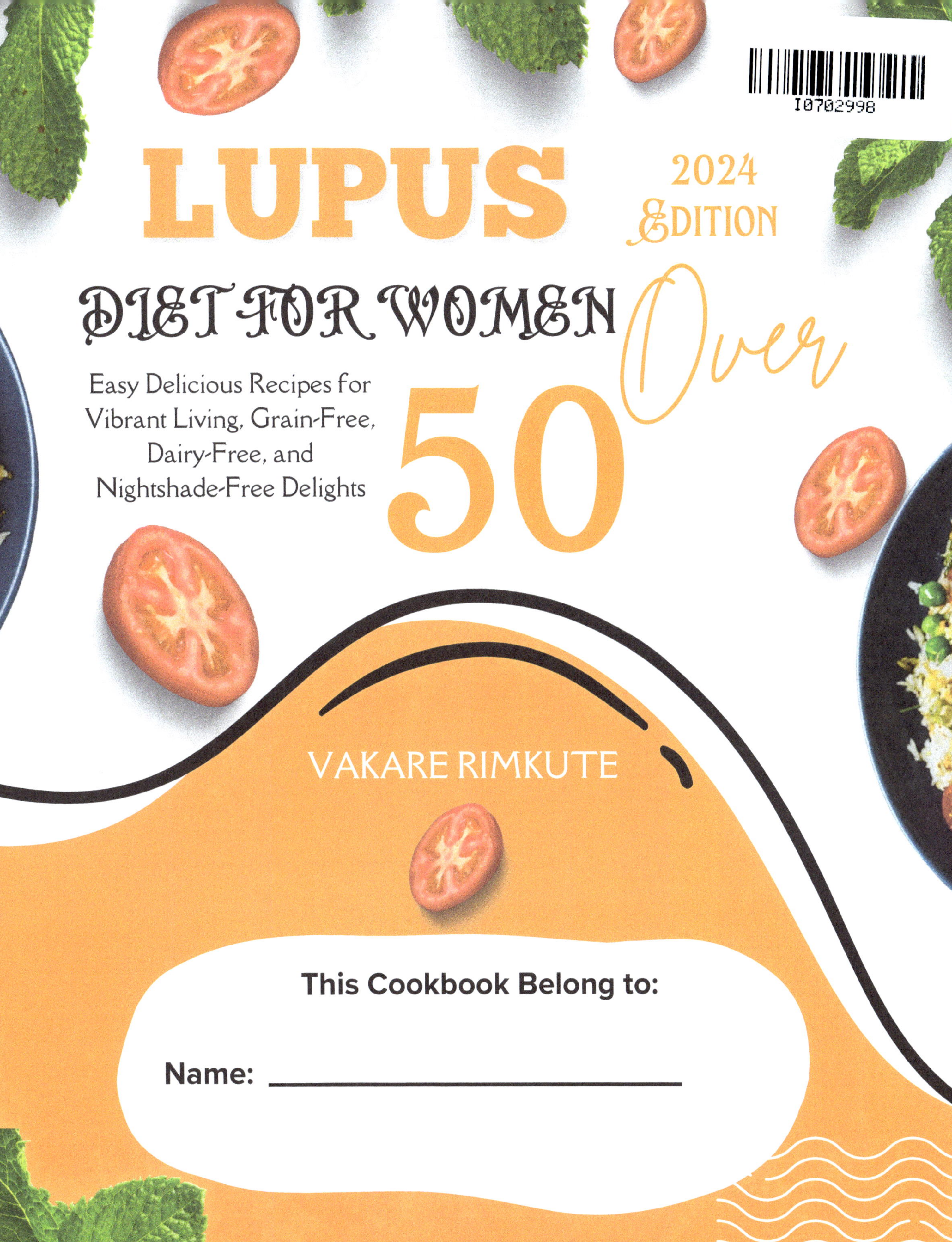

LUPUS
2024 EDITION
DIET FOR WOMEN
Over
Easy Delicious Recipes for Vibrant Living, Grain-Free, Dairy-Free, and Nightshade-Free Delights
50
VAKARE RIMKUTE
This Cookbook Belong to:
Name: _______________________

Copyright © 2024 by Vakare Rimkute

⚠ Disclaimer

The recipes and information presented in this cookbook are intended for general informational purposes only. While Vakare Rimkute has made every effort to ensure the accuracy and completeness of the content, they make no representations or warranties of any kind, express or implied, about the suitability or applicability of the recipes for any purpose .

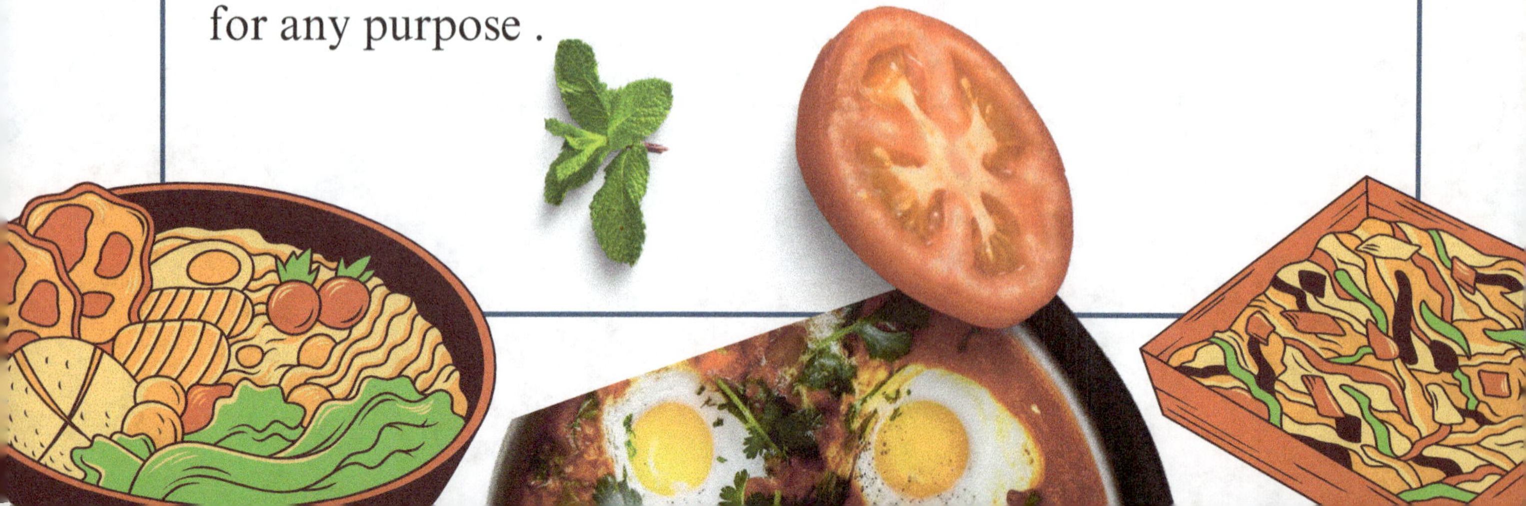

Introduction to the Lupus Diet for Women Over 50

Understanding Lupus

Living with lupus presents unique challenges, especially for women over 50. Lupus is a chronic autoimmune disease where the immune system mistakenly attacks healthy tissues, leading to inflammation, pain, and damage to various parts of the body. While there is no cure for lupus, proper management of the condition can significantly improve quality of life. One of the most effective ways to manage lupus is through diet.

Lupus can affect multiple organs and systems in the body, including the skin, joints, kidneys, heart, lungs, and brain. Symptoms can vary widely but often include fatigue, joint pain, skin rashes, and fever. The disease is characterized by periods of flares (when symptoms worsen) and remissions (when symptoms improve).

Why Diet Matters

Diet plays a crucial role in managing lupus symptoms and overall health. For women over 50, maintaining a balanced, nutrient-rich diet is even more critical due to age-related changes such as decreased bone density, changes in metabolism, and increased risk of cardiovascular disease.

- **Reducing Inflammation**: Certain foods can help reduce inflammation, a key concern for lupus patients. Anti-inflammatory foods can help manage pain and swelling.
- **Boosting Immune Function**: Proper nutrition supports a healthy immune system, which is essential for those with autoimmune diseases.
- **Maintaining Healthy Weight**: Managing weight through diet can reduce the risk of comorbidities like cardiovascular disease and diabetes, which are more common in lupus patients.

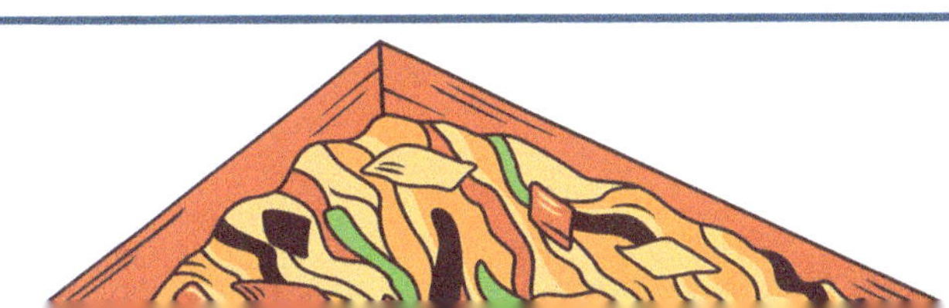

How to Use This Cookbook

This cookbook is designed to guide you through the principles of a lupus-friendly diet, offering practical advice and delicious recipes tailored to the unique needs of women over 50. Here's how to make the most of it:

- **Understanding Nutritional Needs**: Learn about the specific dietary requirements for women over 50 with lupus, including key nutrients and foods to avoid.
- **Exploring Recipes:** Dive into a variety of recipes categorized by meal type (breakfast, lunch, dinner, snacks, desserts, and beverages). Each recipe is designed to be nutritious, easy to prepare, and delicious.
- **Using Recipe Symbols:** Look for symbols indicating gluten-free, dairy-free, low-sodium, and other special dietary considerations to find recipes that meet your specific needs.
- **Meal Planning**: Utilize sample meal plans and tips for meal prepping to make healthy eating easier and more consistent.
- **Healthy Substitutions**: Discover alternatives for common inflammatory foods and ingredients, making it simpler to stick to a lupus-friendly diet.
- **Nutritional Information:** Each recipe includes nutritional information to help you keep track of your intake of essential nutrients.

Personal Note from the Author

As someone who understands the challenges of living with lupus, I have crafted this cookbook to provide you with the tools and knowledge needed to make informed dietary choices. I hope these recipes inspire you to create meals that not only support your health but also bring joy to your table. Remember, managing lupus is a journey, and every positive dietary change you make is a step towards better health and well-being.

How Lupus Affects Women Over 50

1. Increased Risk of Osteoporosis

- **Why It Happens:** Women over 50 are at increased risk of osteoporosis due to hormonal changes associated with menopause. Lupus and the use of corticosteroids, commonly prescribed for lupus management, further exacerbate this risk by reducing bone density.
- **Impact**: Higher likelihood of fractures and bone pain, necessitating a focus on bone health through diet and lifestyle.

2. Cardiovascular Health

- **Why It Happens**: Lupus increases the risk of cardiovascular disease, which is already a concern as women age. Inflammation from lupus, coupled with traditional risk factors like high blood pressure and cholesterol, contributes to this heightened risk.
- **Impact**: Greater incidence of heart attacks, strokes, and other cardiovascular issues, requiring vigilant management of heart health through diet, exercise, and medical care.

3. Joint Pain and Mobility Issues

- **Why It Happens:** Joint pain and arthritis are common in lupus patients. For women over 50, age-related wear and tear on the joints can compound these symptoms, leading to increased pain and reduced mobility.
- **Impact**: Difficulty in performing daily activities, which can affect independence and quality of life. Physical therapy and a diet rich in anti-inflammatory foods can help manage symptoms.

4. Kidney Function

- **Why It Happens:** Lupus nephritis, an inflammation of the kidneys caused by lupus, can impair kidney function. Aging naturally reduces kidney efficiency, making older women more vulnerable.
- **Impact**: Need for regular monitoring of kidney function and a diet low in sodium and high in hydration to support kidney health.

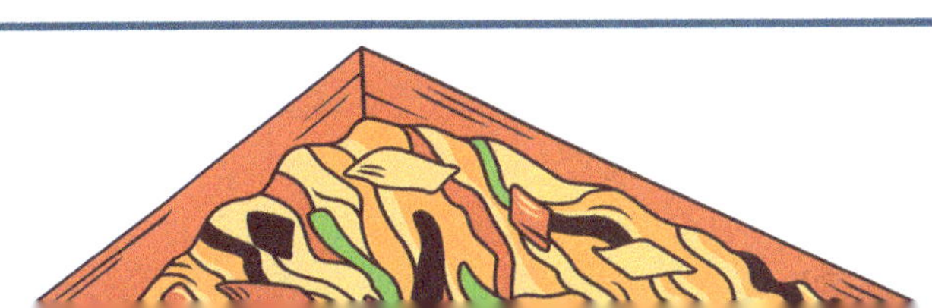

How Lupus Affects Women Over 50

5. Cognitive Function

- **Why It Happens:** Lupus can affect the central nervous system, leading to cognitive issues such as memory problems, confusion, and difficulty concentrating. Age-related cognitive decline can exacerbate these symptoms.
- **Impact**: Challenges in maintaining mental clarity and cognitive function, emphasizing the importance of a nutrient-rich diet and mental exercises to support brain health.

6. Skin and Hair

- **Why It Happens**: Lupus can cause skin rashes, lesions, and hair loss. Aging skin is more susceptible to damage and slower to heal.
- **Impact**: Increased need for skin care and protection, as well as dietary support for healthy skin and hair.

7. Fatigue and Energy Levels

- **Why It Happens:** Chronic fatigue is a hallmark of lupus, and it can be more pronounced in older women due to decreased energy reserves and slower recovery times.
- **Impact**: Persistent tiredness affecting daily activities and overall well-being, making it essential to manage energy levels through proper nutrition, sleep, and stress management.

8. Emotional and Mental Health

- **Why It Happens:** Living with a chronic illness like lupus can lead to depression, anxiety, and stress. These issues can be more significant in older women who may also be coping with other age-related changes and losses.
- **Impact**: Greater need for emotional support and mental health care, including counseling, social support, and mindfulness practices.

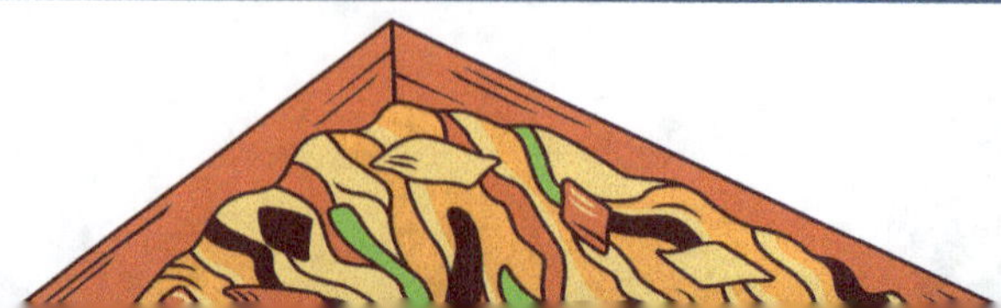

TABLE OF

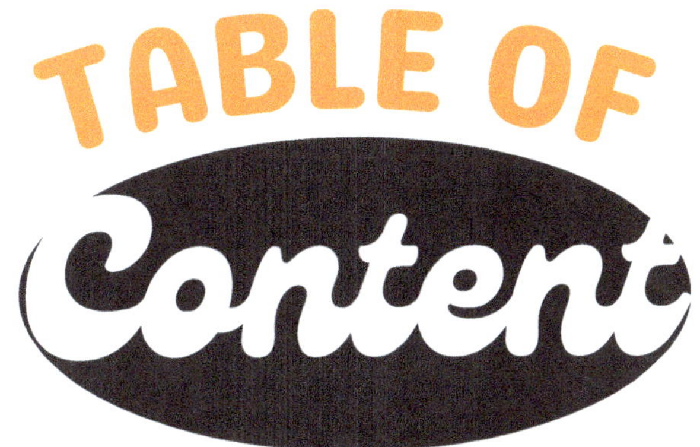

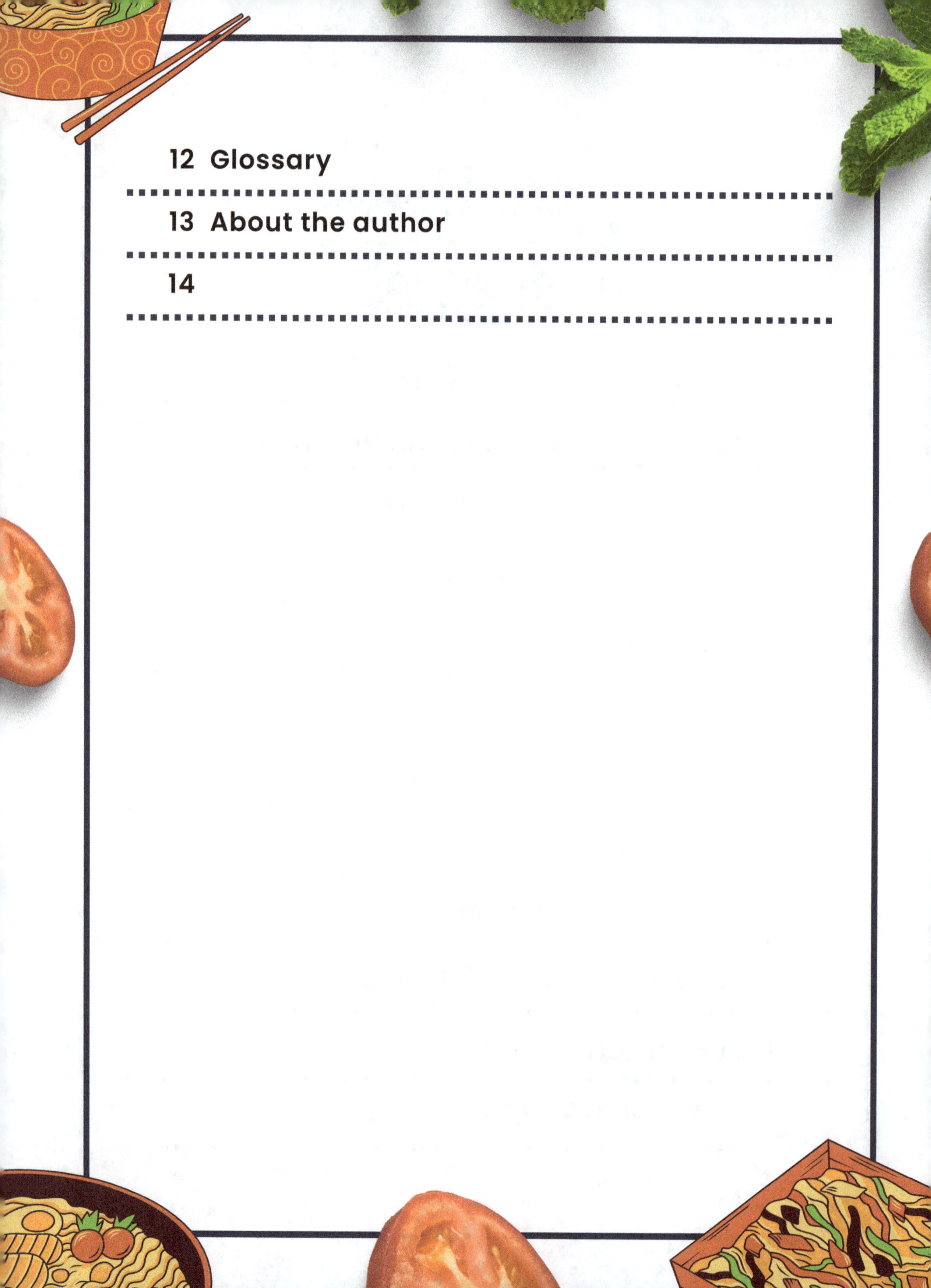

CHAPTER 1

Understanding Lupus and Nutrition

What is Lupus?

Lupus is a chronic autoimmune illness, officially known as systemic lupus erythematosus (SLE). In autoimmune disorders, the immune system, which is supposed to protect the body from infections and external invaders, erroneously assaults healthy tissues. Lupus can affect several organs and systems in the body, causing various symptoms.

Types of Lupus

- **Cutaneous Lupus Erythematosus:** Affects only the skin, causing rashes and lesions.
- **Drug-Induced Lupus:** Triggered by certain prescription medications, with symptoms similar to SLE but typically resolving once the medication is stopped.
- **Neonatal Lupus:** A rare condition affecting newborns, caused by antibodies from the mother.

Symptoms of Lupus

1. **Fatigue:** Extreme tiredness that doesn't improve with rest.
2. **Joint Pain and Swelling:** Often affecting the hands, wrists, and knees.
3. **Skin Rashes:** Including a characteristic "butterfly-shaped" rash across the cheeks and nose.
4. **Photosensitivity:** Sensitivity to sunlight, causing rashes or worsening symptoms.
5. **Fever:** Low-grade fevers that come and go.
6. **Hair Loss:** Thinning hair or bald spots.
7. **Raynaud's Phenomenon:** Fingers and toes turning white or blue in response to cold or stress.
8. **Kidney Problems:** Inflammation of the kidneys (lupus nephritis), which can lead to kidney failure if untreated.

Challenges of Living with Lupus

- **Fluctuating Symptoms:**
Lupus is characterized by periods of flares (when symptoms worsen) and remissions (when symptoms improve or disappear). This unpredictability can make planning and managing daily life difficult.

- **Chronic Pain:**
Persistent pain from joint inflammation, muscle aches, and headaches can significantly impact quality of life.

- **Fatigue**:
Severe and persistent fatigue can interfere with work, social activities, and self-care.

- **Emotional and Mental Health:**
Dealing with a chronic illness can lead to anxiety, depression, and feelings of isolation. Cognitive symptoms like memory loss and difficulty concentrating (often referred to as "lupus fog") can also be challenging.

- **Physical Appearance:**
Skin rashes, hair loss, and weight changes can affect self-esteem and body image.

- **Sensitivity to Sunlight:**
Many people with lupus need to avoid direct sunlight, which can limit outdoor activities and social interactions.

- **Medication Side Effects:**
Long-term use of medications, especially corticosteroids, can lead to side effects such as weight gain, osteoporosis, high blood pressure, and increased risk of infections.

- **Impact on Organs:**
Lupus can affect major organs, leading to serious conditions such as kidney disease, cardiovascular problems, and lung issues.

- **Social and Work Limitations:**
Frequent medical appointments, hospitalizations, and the need for rest can impact professional life and social relationships.

- **Financial Strain:**
The cost of ongoing medical care, medications, and possible loss of income due to inability to work can cause financial stress.

Causes of Lupus

Genetic Factors

- **Family History:** Individuals with a family history of lupus or other autoimmune diseases have a higher risk of developing lupus.
- **Genetic Predisposition**: Certain genes are associated with an increased risk of lupus. However, having these genes does not guarantee that an individual will develop the disease, indicating that genetics alone are not sufficient to cause lupus.

Environmental Triggers

- **Infections**: Certain viral and bacterial infections can trigger lupus or cause flare-ups in people who are genetically predisposed. For example, the Epstein-Barr virus (which causes mononucleosis) has been linked to an increased risk of lupus.
- **Sunlight (UV Radiation)**: Exposure to ultraviolet (UV) light can trigger skin lesions and internal disease flares in individuals with lupus.
- **Medications**: Some drugs, such as certain antibiotics, blood pressure medications, and anti-seizure medications, can induce lupus-like symptoms.

Hormonal Factors

- **Sex Hormones:** The higher prevalence of lupus in women, especially during their childbearing years, suggests that hormones such as estrogen play a role in the disease. Hormonal fluctuations during menstrual cycles, pregnancy, and menopause can also affect lupus activity.
- **Prolactin:** Some studies suggest that the hormone prolactin, which is higher in women and increases during pregnancy, may play a role in lupus.

Immune System Abnormalities

- **Autoimmunity**: Lupus is characterized by the immune system mistakenly attacking healthy tissues. Abnormalities in immune system regulation and response can contribute to the development of lupus.
- **Antibody Production:** People with lupus often produce abnormal antibodies that target their own tissues, leading to inflammation and tissue damage.

Nutritional Needs for Women Over 50

1. Calcium and Vitamin D

- **Importance**: Essential for maintaining bone health and reducing the risk of osteoporosis, which becomes more prevalent after menopause.
- **Sources**: Dairy products (milk, cheese, yogurt), fortified plant-based milks (almond, soy), leafy green vegetables (kale, collard greens), and fortified cereals.
- **Vitamin D Sources:** Sun exposure, fatty fish (salmon, mackerel), fortified foods, and supplements if necessary.

2. Protein

- **Importance**: Helps maintain muscle mass, supports immune function, and aids in tissue repair, which is particularly important for those with lupus.
- **Sources**: Lean meats (chicken, turkey), fish, eggs, dairy products, legumes (beans, lentils), nuts, seeds, and plant-based proteins (tofu, tempeh).

3. Omega-3 Fatty Acids

- **Importance**: Anti-inflammatory properties that can help manage lupus symptoms and support heart health.
- **Sources**: Fatty fish (salmon, sardines, mackerel), flaxseeds, chia seeds, walnuts, and omega-3 supplements (fish oil or algae oil).

4. Fiber

- **Importance**: Promotes digestive health, helps control blood sugar levels, and supports heart health.
- **Sources**: Whole grains (oats, quinoa, brown rice), fruits (berries, apples, pears), vegetables (broccoli, carrots, leafy greens), legumes, nuts, and seeds.

5. Antioxidants

- **Importance**: Help protect cells from damage caused by inflammation and oxidative stress, which is beneficial for managing lupus.
- **Sources**: Fruits and vegetables rich in vitamins A, C, and E (berries, citrus fruits, peppers, spinach, sweet potatoes), nuts, seeds, and green tea.

6. Iron

- **Importance**: Necessary for maintaining healthy blood cells and preventing anemia, which can be a concern for women with lupus.
- **Sources**: Lean meats, fish, poultry, beans, lentils, tofu, fortified cereals, and dark leafy greens. Pairing iron-rich foods with vitamin C sources (citrus fruits, tomatoes) can enhance absorption.

7. Magnesium

- **Importance**: Supports muscle and nerve function, bone health, and energy production.
- **Sources**: Nuts (almonds, cashews), seeds (pumpkin, sunflower), whole grains, legumes, leafy green vegetables, and dark chocolate.

8. B Vitamins

- **Importance**: Essential for energy production, brain health, and red blood cell formation.
- **Sources**: Whole grains, meat, eggs, dairy products, legumes, leafy greens, nuts, and seeds.

9. Hydration

- **Importance**: Maintaining adequate hydration is crucial for overall health and can help manage some symptoms of lupus.
- **Sources**: Water, herbal teas, and water-rich foods (fruits and vegetables).

10. Low Sodium

- **Importance**: Helps manage blood pressure and reduce the risk of heart disease, which is important for women with lupus who may have an increased risk of cardiovascular issues.
- **Sources**: Focus on fresh, unprocessed foods, use herbs and spices for flavor instead of salt, and read food labels to avoid high-sodium processed foods.

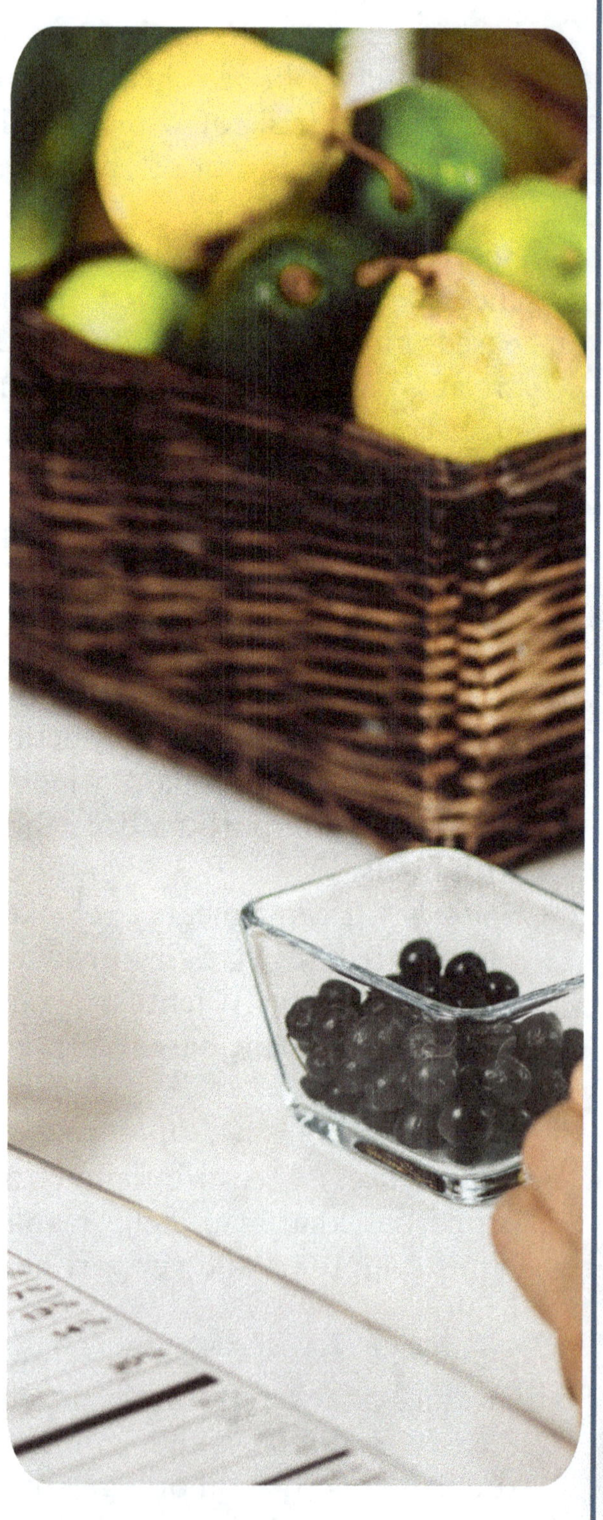

Foods to Avoid with Lupus

1. Processed Foods

- **Why Avoid:** Processed foods often contain high levels of unhealthy fats, sugars, and additives that can increase inflammation.
- **Examples**: Packaged snacks, fast food, frozen dinners, and processed meats (like hot dogs and deli meats).

2. Sugary Foods and Beverages

- **Why Avoid:** High sugar intake can lead to weight gain and increased inflammation, exacerbating lupus symptoms.
- **Examples**: Sodas, candies, pastries, and other desserts with high sugar content.

3. High-Sodium Foods

- **Why Avoid**: Excessive sodium can lead to high blood pressure and fluid retention, both of which are concerns for lupus patients, particularly those on corticosteroids.
- **Examples**: Canned soups, salty snacks, processed foods, and restaurant meals.

4. Saturated and Trans Fats

- **Why Avoid**: These fats can contribute to inflammation and increase the risk of heart disease, which lupus patients are already at higher risk for.
- **Examples**: Fried foods, baked goods made with hydrogenated oils, fatty cuts of meat, and full-fat dairy products.

5. Alcohol

- **Why Avoid**: Alcohol can interfere with lupus medications and exacerbate liver issues, which are more common in lupus patients.
- **Examples**: Beer, wine, spirits, and mixed alcoholic drinks.

6. Nightshade Vegetables

- **Why Avoid**: Some people with lupus report increased inflammation and joint pain after consuming nightshade vegetables, though this is not universally experienced.
- **Examples**: Tomatoes, potatoes, eggplants, and bell peppers.

7. Gluten

- **Why Avoid**: While not all lupus patients are sensitive to gluten, some may have celiac disease or gluten intolerance, which can exacerbate symptoms.
- **Examples**: Wheat, barley, rye, and foods made with these grains like bread, pasta, and baked goods.

8. Alfalfa Sprouts

- **Why Avoid:** Alfalfa sprouts contain an amino acid called L-canavanine that can stimulate the immune system and potentially trigger lupus flares.
- **Examples**: Alfalfa sprouts in salads, sandwiches, and smoothies.

9. Garlic and Echinacea

- **Why Avoid**: Both garlic and echinacea are known to boost the immune system, which might seem beneficial, but for lupus patients, this can potentially lead to an overactive immune response.
- **Examples**: Raw garlic, garlic supplements, echinacea tea, and supplements.

10. Caffeine

- **Why Avoid**: Excessive caffeine can contribute to increased stress and anxiety, which can trigger lupus flares.
- **Examples**: Coffee, energy drinks, certain teas, and sodas.

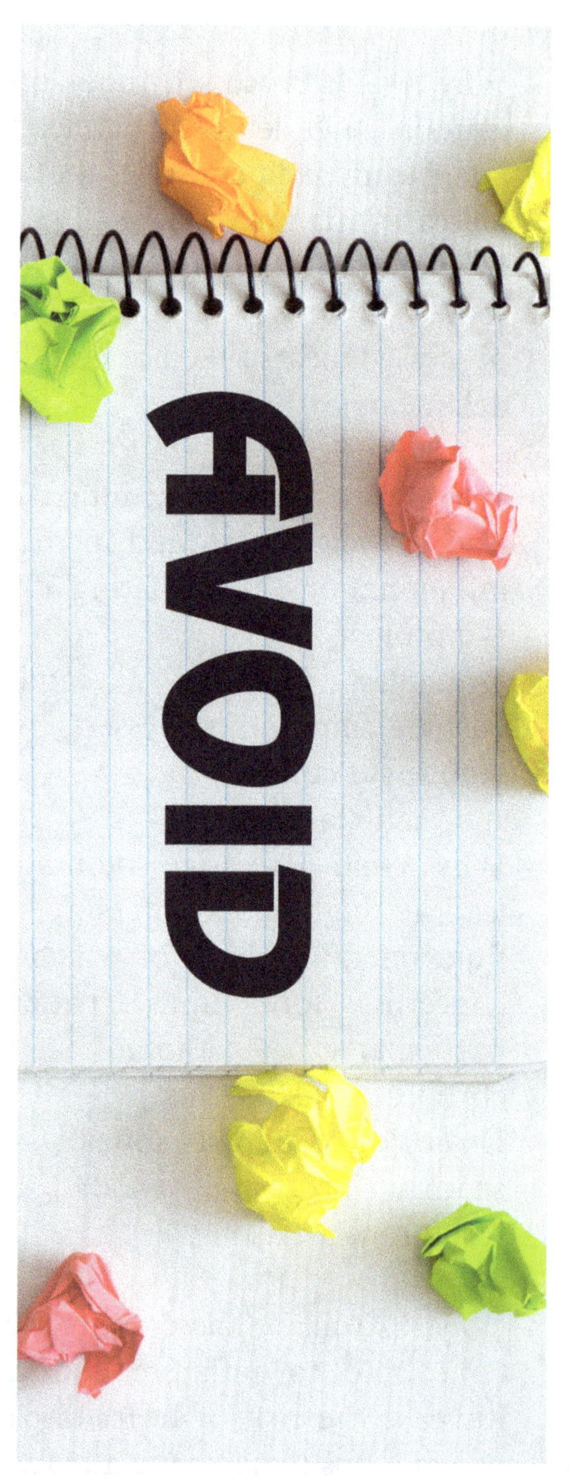

Beneficial Foods for Lupus Management

Anti-inflammatory Foods

Fruits

- **Berries**: Blueberries, strawberries, raspberries, and blackberries are rich in antioxidants and anti-inflammatory compounds.
- **Citrus Fruits:** Oranges, lemons, and grapefruits provide vitamin C, which has anti-inflammatory properties.
- **Other Fruits:** Apples, cherries, and pineapples are also beneficial.

Vegetables

- **Leafy Greens**: Spinach, kale, and Swiss chard are packed with vitamins and antioxidants that help reduce inflammation.
- **Cruciferous Vegetables**: Broccoli, cauliflower, Brussels sprouts, and cabbage contain sulforaphane, which has anti-inflammatory effects.
- **Other Veggies:** Bell peppers, carrots, and beets are rich in vitamins and minerals that combat inflammation.

Whole Grains

- **Quinoa**: High in protein and fiber, quinoa is a great anti-inflammatory grain.
- **Brown Rice:** A good source of fiber and antioxidants.
- **Oats**: Contains avenanthramides, which have anti-inflammatory properties.

Healthy Fats

- **Olive Oil:** Rich in monounsaturated fats and oleocanthal, which have anti-inflammatory effects.
- **Avocados**: Contain healthy fats, fiber, and anti-inflammatory compounds.
- **Nuts and Seeds:** Almonds, walnuts, chia seeds, and flaxseeds are high in omega-3 fatty acids, which reduce inflammation.

Fatty Fish

- **Examples**: Salmon, mackerel, sardines, and trout are excellent sources of omega-3 fatty acids that help reduce inflammation.

Legumes

- **Examples**: Lentils, chickpeas, black beans, and kidney beans are high in fiber, protein, and antioxidants.

Spices and Herbs

- **Turmeric**: Contains curcumin, a potent anti-inflammatory compound.
- **Ginger**: Has anti-inflammatory and antioxidant properties.
- **Garlic**: Though it can be a trigger for some, it also has strong anti-inflammatory effects for many people.

Beneficial Foods for Lupus Management

Superfoods for Lupus

Berries

- **Why They're Super:** High in antioxidants like anthocyanins and vitamin C, which help reduce oxidative stress and inflammation.

Fatty Fish

- **Why They're Super**: High in omega-3 fatty acids, which have been shown to reduce inflammation and improve cardiovascular health.

Leafy Greens

- **Why They're Super**: Packed with vitamins A, C, and K, and minerals like calcium and iron, which support overall health and reduce inflammation.

Turmeric

- **Why It's Super:** Curcumin, the active compound in turmeric, is a powerful anti-inflammatory and antioxidant.

Ginger

- **Why It's Super:** Contains gingerol, which has potent anti-inflammatory and antioxidant effects.

Chia Seeds

- **Why They're Super**: High in omega-3 fatty acids, fiber, and protein, which help reduce inflammation and support overall health.

Flaxseeds

- **Why They're Super:** Rich in alpha-linolenic acid (ALA), a type of omega-3 fatty acid, and lignans, which have antioxidant properties.

Quinoa

- **Why It's Super:** A complete protein source with all nine essential amino acids, high in fiber and antioxidants.

Green Tea

- **Why It's Super**: Contains EGCG, which reduces inflammation and protects cells from damage.

Avocado

- **Why It's Super**: Rich in monounsaturated fats, fiber, vitamins, and minerals that support heart health and reduce inflammation.

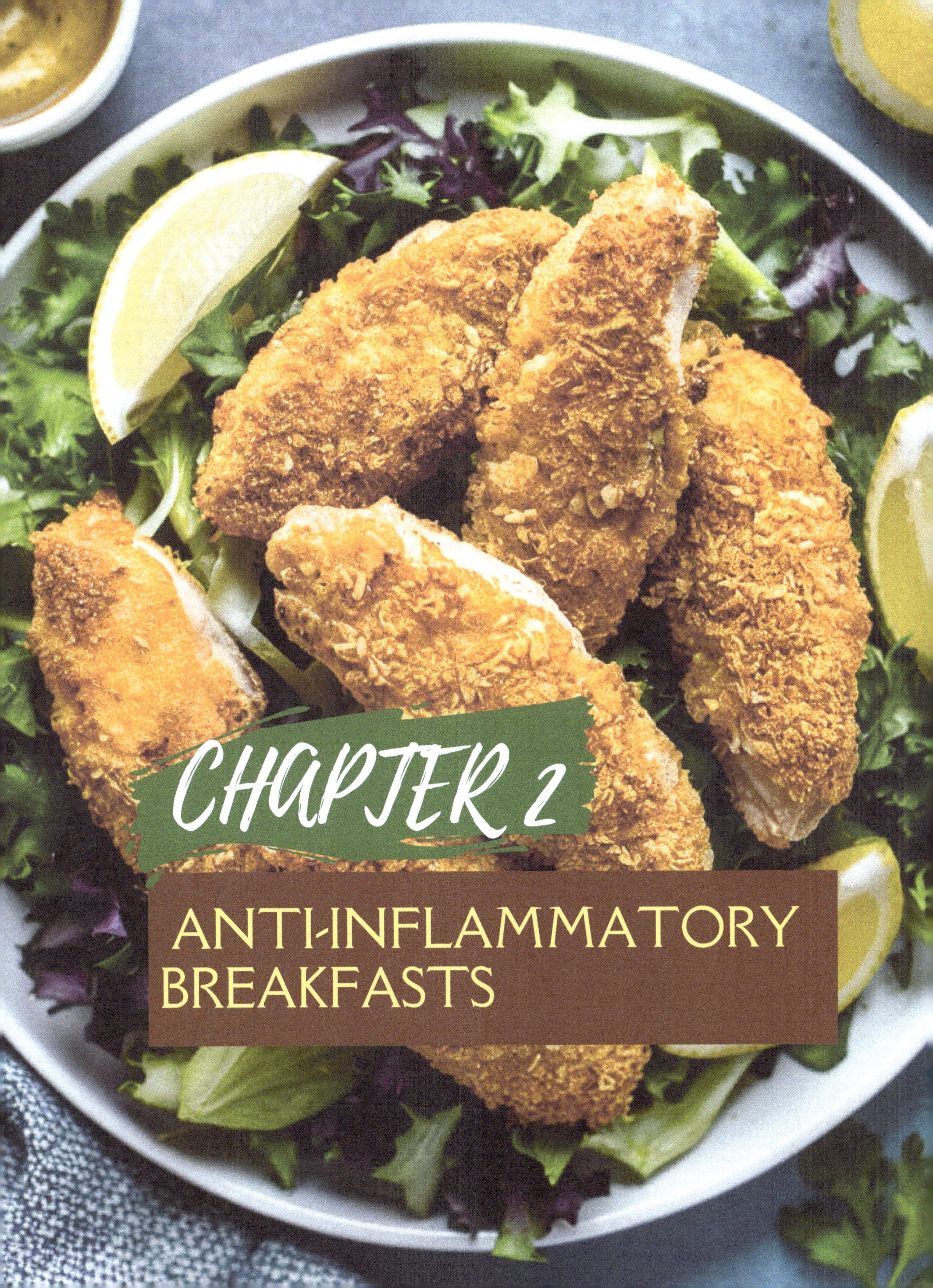

CHAPTER 2
ANTI-INFLAMMATORY BREAKFASTS

SPINACH AND MUSHROOM FRITTATA

Ingredients

- 1 cup fresh spinach, chopped
- 1 cup mushrooms, sliced
- 6 large eggs
- 1/4 cup milk (dairy or non-dairy)
- 1/2 cup shredded cheese (optional, can use dairy-free cheese)
- 1 small onion, finely chopped
- 1 clove garlic, minced
- Salt and pepper to taste
- 1 tablespoon olive oil

Instructions

- Preheat your oven to 375°F (190°C).
- In a large oven-safe skillet, heat the olive oil over medium heat.
- Add the chopped onion and garlic, sauté until fragrant and the onion is translucent, about 2-3 minutes.
- Add the sliced mushrooms to the skillet, cook until they release their moisture and start to brown, about 5 minutes.
- Add the chopped spinach to the skillet and cook until wilted, about 1-2 minutes.
- In a mixing bowl, whisk together the eggs, milk, salt, and pepper.
- Pour the egg mixture over the vegetables in the skillet. If using, sprinkle the shredded cheese evenly over the top.
- Cook on the stove for about 2-3 minutes until the edges start to set.
- Transfer the skillet to the preheated oven and bake for 10-12 minutes, or until the frittata is fully set and lightly golden on top.
- Remove from the oven, let it cool slightly, then slice into wedges and serve.

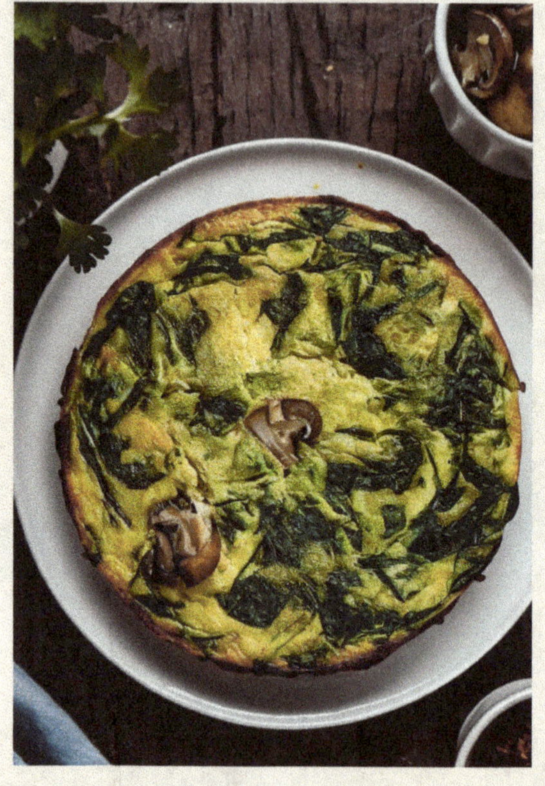

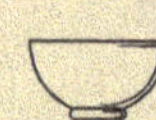 **Preparation Time : 10 min**

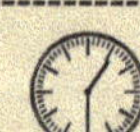 **Total Time : 25 min**

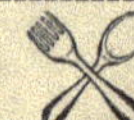 **Servings : 4**

Nutritional Info

- Calories: 180
- Protein: 12g
- Fat: 12g
- Carbohydrates: 5g
- Fiber: 1g

SWEET POTATO AND KALE HASH

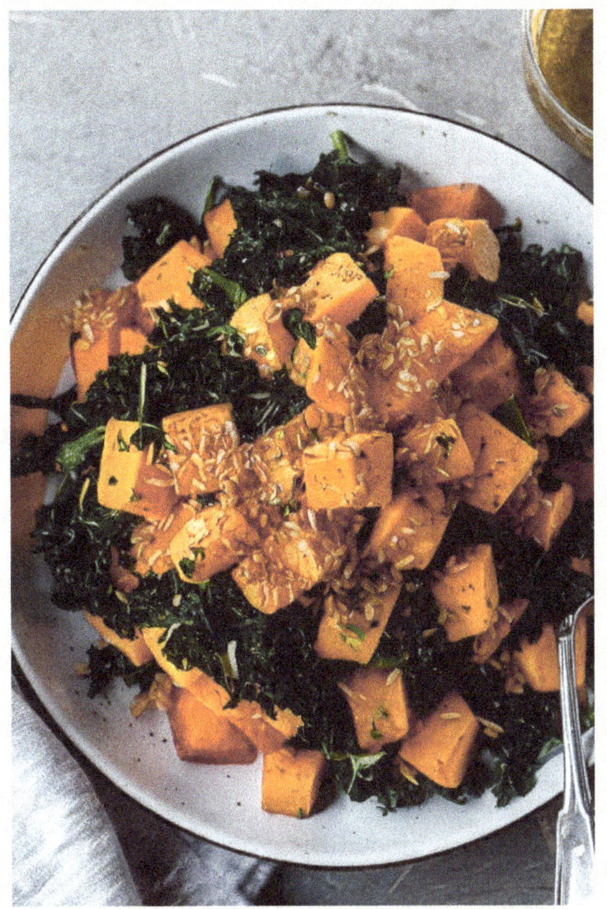

Ingredients

- 2 medium sweet potatoes, peeled and diced
- 1 bunch kale, stems removed and leaves chopped
- 1 onion, diced
- 2 garlic cloves, minced
- 1 tablespoon olive oil
- Salt and pepper, to taste

Instructions

- Heat olive oil in a large skillet over medium heat.
- Add onion and garlic, and sauté until onion is translucent.
- Add sweet potatoes and cook, stirring occasionally, until they start to soften, about 10 minutes.
- Stir in kale and cook until wilted.
- Season with salt and pepper.
- Serve hot.

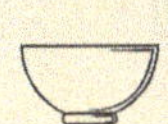 **Preparation Time : 10 min**

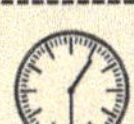 **Total Time : 30 min**

 **Servings : 4**

Nutritional Info

- Calories: 180
- Fat: 4g
- Carbohydrates: 35g
- Fiber: 5g
- Protein: 3g

AVOCADO TOAST WITH POACHED EGG

Ingredients

- 1 slice of whole grain bread
- 1/2 ripe avocado
- 1 egg
- Salt and pepper to taste
- Optional toppings: red pepper flakes, chopped chives.

Instructions

- Fill a small saucepan with water and bring it to a simmer.
- Crack the egg into a small bowl or cup.
- Create a gentle whirlpool in the water and carefully slide the egg into the center.
- Cook for about 3-4 minutes for a soft yolk, or longer for a firmer yolk.
- Remove the egg with a slotted spoon and place it on a paper towel to drain.
- While the egg is poaching, cut the avocado in half and remove the pit.
- Scoop out the flesh into a bowl and mash it with a fork.
- Toast the bread until golden brown and crispy.
- Spread the mashed avocado evenly onto the toasted bread.
- Place the poached egg on top.
- Season with additional salt and pepper if desired.
- Add any optional toppings like red pepper flakes, chopped chives, or a squeeze of lemon juice.
- Serve the avocado toast immediately and enjoy!

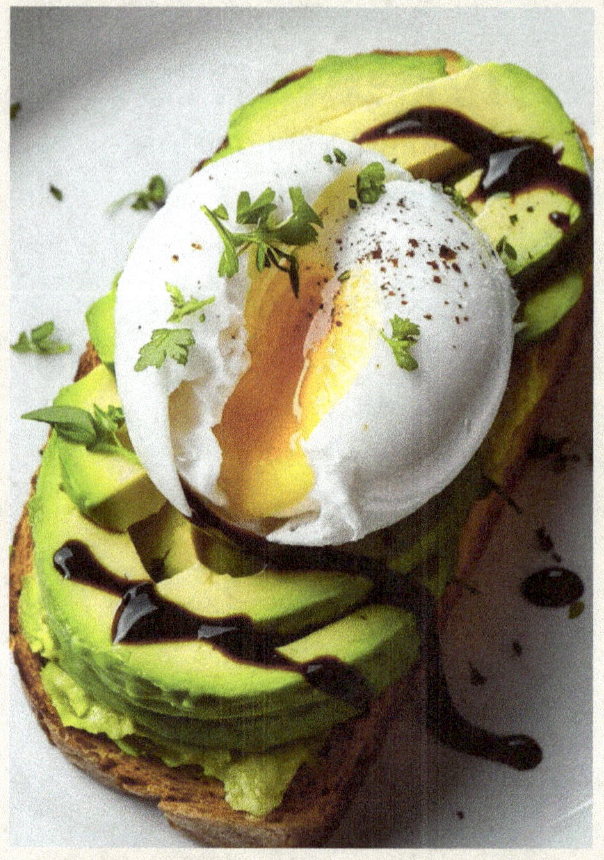

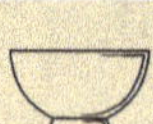 **Preparation Time : 5 min**

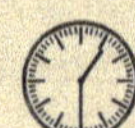 **Total Time : 10 min**

 **Servings : 1**

Nutritional Info

- Calories: 300 kcal
- Protein: 10g
- Fat: 20g
- Carbohydrates: 25g
- Fiber: 10g

TURMERIC AND GINGER SMOOTHIE

Ingredients

- 1 ripe banana
- 1 cup coconut milk (or any milk of your choice)
- 1/2 teaspoon ground turmeric
- 1/2 teaspoon grated ginger
- 1 tablespoon honey (optional, adjust to taste)
- Handful of ice cubes

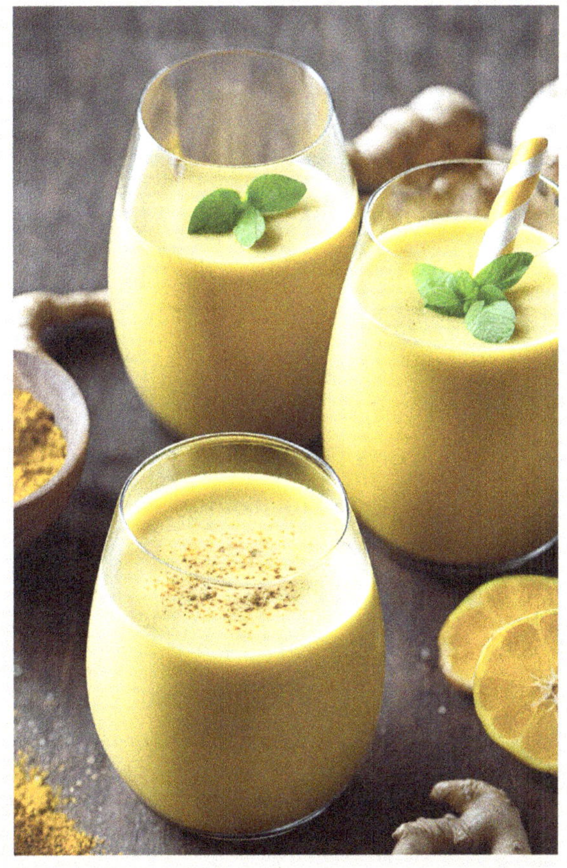

Instructions

- Peel and chop the banana.
- Add all ingredients to a blender.
- Blend until smooth and creamy.
- Taste and adjust sweetness if necessary by adding more honey.
- Serve immediately in glasses.

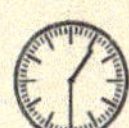 **Preparation Time : 5 min**

 **Total Time : 5 min**

Servings : 2

Nutritional Info

- Calories: 120 kcal
- Fat: 6g
- Carbohydrates: 20g
- Protein: 1g
- Fiber: 3g

CHIA SEED BREAKFAST PUDDING

Ingredients

- 2 tablespoons chia seeds
- 1/2 cup almond milk (or any milk of your choice)
- 1/2 teaspoon vanilla extract
- 1 tablespoon honey or maple syrup (optional)
- Fresh fruits (such as berries, sliced banana, or mango) for topping
- Nuts or seeds for topping (such as sliced almonds, chopped walnuts, or pumpkin seeds)

Instructions

- In a bowl or jar, combine chia seeds, almond milk, vanilla extract, and honey or maple syrup (if using). Stir well to combine.
- Cover the bowl or jar and refrigerate overnight, or for at least 4 hours, to allow the chia seeds to absorb the liquid and thicken into a pudding-like consistency.
- Once the chia seed pudding has thickened, give it a good stir.
- Serve the chia seed pudding chilled, topped with your favorite fruits, nuts, or seeds.
- Enjoy your nutritious and delicious Chia Seed Breakfast Pudding!

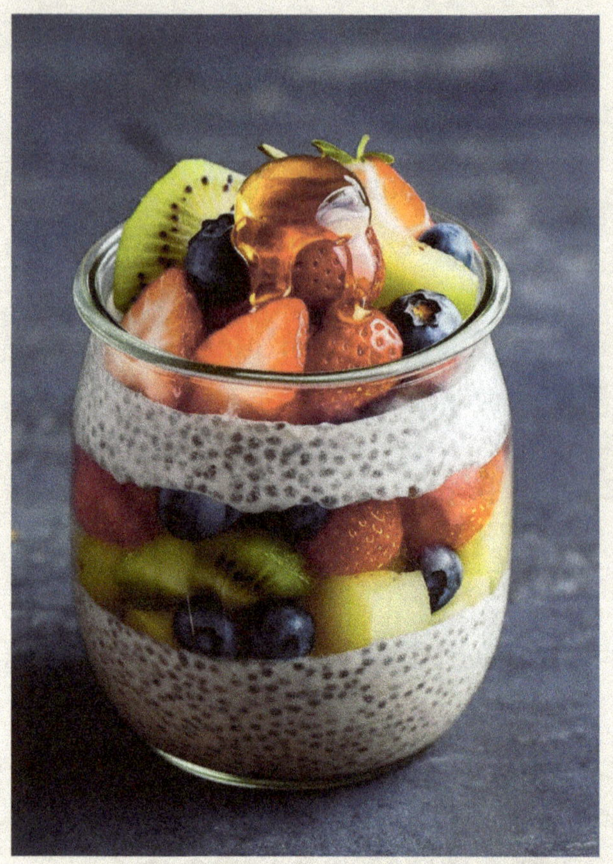

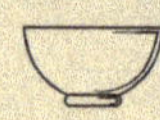 **Preparation Time : 5 min**

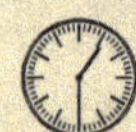 **Total Time : 0 min**

 **Servings : 1**

Nutritional Info

- Calories: 220 kcal
- Protein: 6g
- Carbohydrates: 20g
- Fat: 14g
- Fiber: 10g

QUINOA AND BERRY BREAKFAST BOWL

Ingredients

- 1 cup quinoa
- 2 cups almond milk (or any milk of your choice)
- 1 tablespoon honey or maple syrup
- 1 teaspoon vanilla extract
- 1 cup mixed berries (strawberries, blueberries, raspberries)
- 1/4 cup chopped nuts (almonds, walnuts, or pecans)
- Optional toppings: sliced bananas, shredded coconut, chia seeds

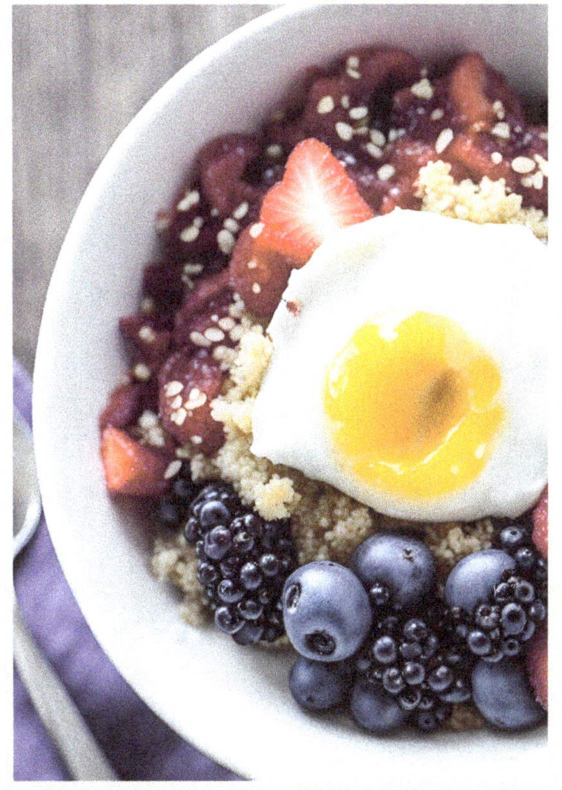

Instructions

1. Rinse quinoa under cold water using a fine mesh strainer.
2. In a medium saucepan, combine quinoa and almond milk. Bring to a boil, then reduce heat to low and simmer for 15-20 minutes, or until quinoa is cooked and liquid is absorbed.
3. Remove from heat and stir in honey or maple syrup and vanilla extract.
4. Divide the cooked quinoa into serving bowls.
5. Top each bowl with mixed berries, chopped nuts, and any other desired toppings.
6. Serve warm or chilled.

Preparation Time : 5 min

Total Time : 20 min

Servings : 2

Nutritional Info

- Calories: 350 kcal
- Protein: 10g
- Carbohydrates: 55g
- Fat: 10g
- Fiber: 8g

BANANA OAT PANCAKES

Ingredients

- 1 ripe banana
- 1/2 cup rolled oats
- 2 eggs
- 1/2 teaspoon cinnamon
- 1/2 teaspoon vanilla extract
- Cooking spray or butter, for cooking
- Optional toppings: fresh berries, maple syrup, Greek yogurt

Instructions

- In a blender, combine the ripe banana, rolled oats, eggs, cinnamon, and vanilla extract. Blend until smooth.
- Heat a non-stick skillet or griddle over medium heat. Lightly coat with cooking spray or melt a small amount of butter.
- Pour the pancake batter onto the skillet, using about 1/4 cup for each pancake. Cook for 2-3 minutes, or until bubbles form on the surface.
- Flip the pancakes and cook for an additional 1-2 minutes, or until golden brown and cooked through.
- Remove the pancakes from the skillet and repeat with the remaining batter. Serve warm with your favorite toppings.

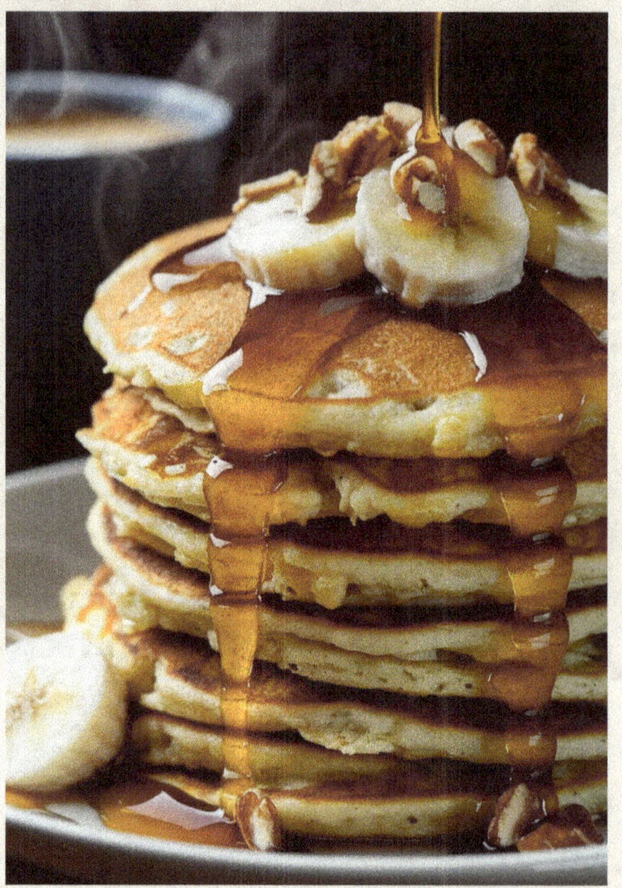

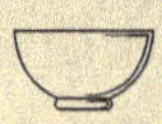 **Preparation Time : 10 min**

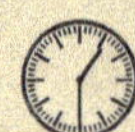 **Total Time : 20 min**

 **Servings : 2**

Nutritional Info

- Calories: 250 kcal
- Protein: 10g
- Carbohydrates: 35g
- Fiber: 5g
- Sugars: 13g
- Fat: 8g

OATMEAL WITH FLAXSEEDS AND WALNUTS

Ingredients

- 1/2 cup rolled oats
- 1 cup water
- 1 tablespoon ground flaxseeds
- 2 tablespoons chopped walnuts
- Optional: honey or maple syrup for sweetness

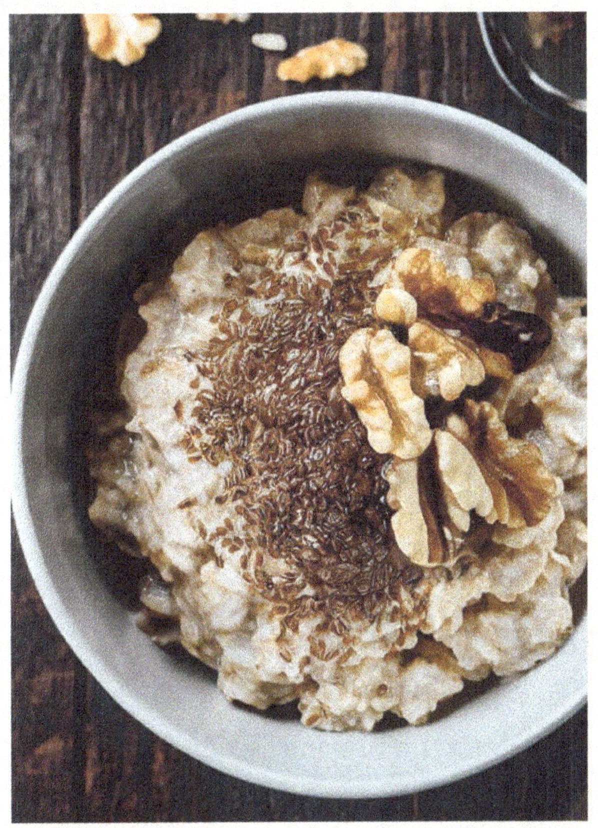

Instructions

- In a small saucepan, bring the water to a boil.
- Stir in the rolled oats and reduce heat to medium-low.
- Cook for about 5 minutes, stirring occasionally, until the oats are tender and creamy.
- Remove from heat and stir in the ground flaxseeds.
- Transfer the oatmeal to a serving bowl and sprinkle with chopped walnuts.
- Drizzle with honey or maple syrup if desired.
- Serve hot and enjoy!

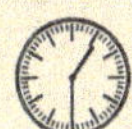 **Preparation Time : 2 min**

 **Total Time : 7 min**

Servings : 1

Nutritional Info

- Calories: 270 kcal
- Protein: 9g
- Carbohydrates: 38g
- Fat: 11g
- Fiber: 7g

GREEK YOGURT PARFAIT WITH FRESH BERRIES

Ingredients

- 1 cup non-fat Greek yogurt
- 1/2 cup fresh strawberries, sliced
- 1/4 cup fresh blueberries
- 1/4 cup fresh raspberries
- 1 tablespoon honey (optional)
- 1/4 cup granola (optional for added texture)

Instructions

- Wash and slice the strawberries.
- Wash the blueberries and raspberries.
- In a glass or bowl, start by adding a layer of Greek yogurt at the bottom.
- Add a layer of sliced strawberries, blueberries, and raspberries on top of the yogurt.
- Drizzle a small amount of honey over the berries if using.
- Add another layer of Greek yogurt on top of the berries.
- Repeat the layers until all ingredients are used, finishing with berries on top.
- Sprinkle granola on top for added texture and crunch, if desired.
- Serve immediately or refrigerate for up to 1 hour to allow flavors to meld.

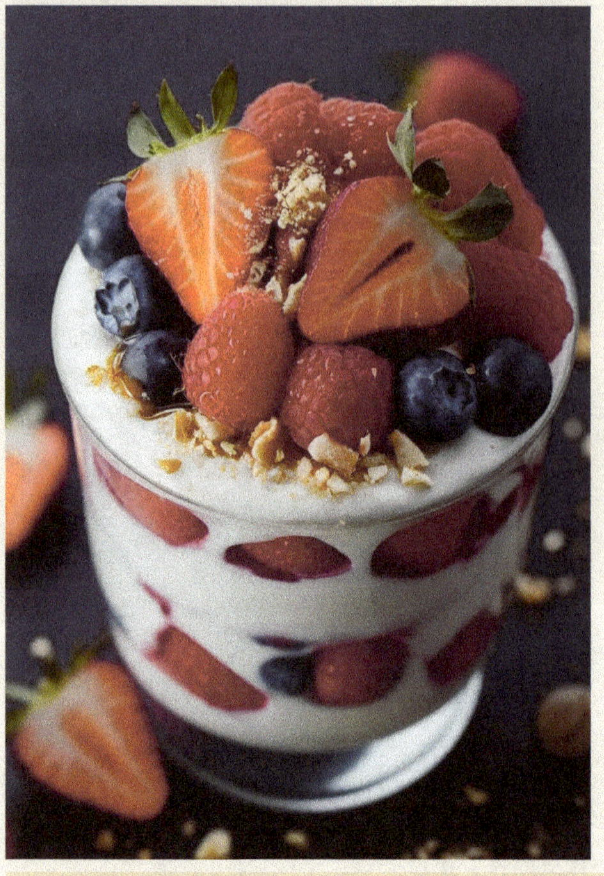

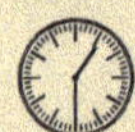 **Preparation Time : 10 min**

 **Total Time : 10 min**

Servings : 1

Nutritional Info

Calories: 150
Protein: 15g
Carbohydrates: 20g
Fat: 2g
Fiber: 4g

Ingredients

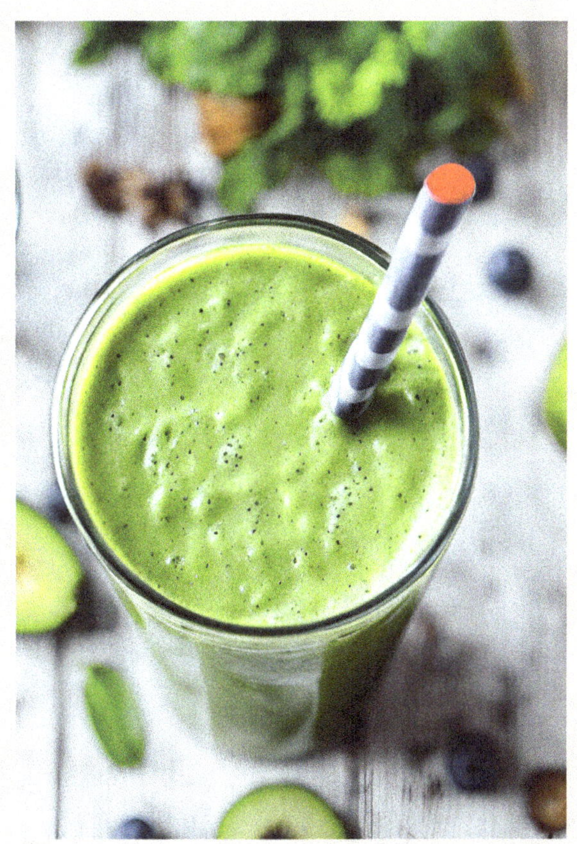

- 1 cup spinach leaves
- 1/2 cucumber, peeled and chopped
- 1/2 green apple, cored and chopped
- 1/2 lemon, juiced
- 1/2 inch fresh ginger, peeled
- 1/2 cup coconut water or plain water
- Ice cubes (optional)

Instructions

- Place all ingredients in a blender.
- Blend until smooth and creamy.
- Add more water if needed to reach desired consistency.
- Pour into a glass and serve immediately.

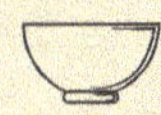 **Preparation Time : 5 min**

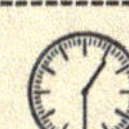 **Total Time : 5 min**

 **Servings : 1**

Nutritional Info

- Calories: 70
- Protein: 2g
- Carbohydrates: 16g
- Fiber: 4g
- Fat: 0.5g

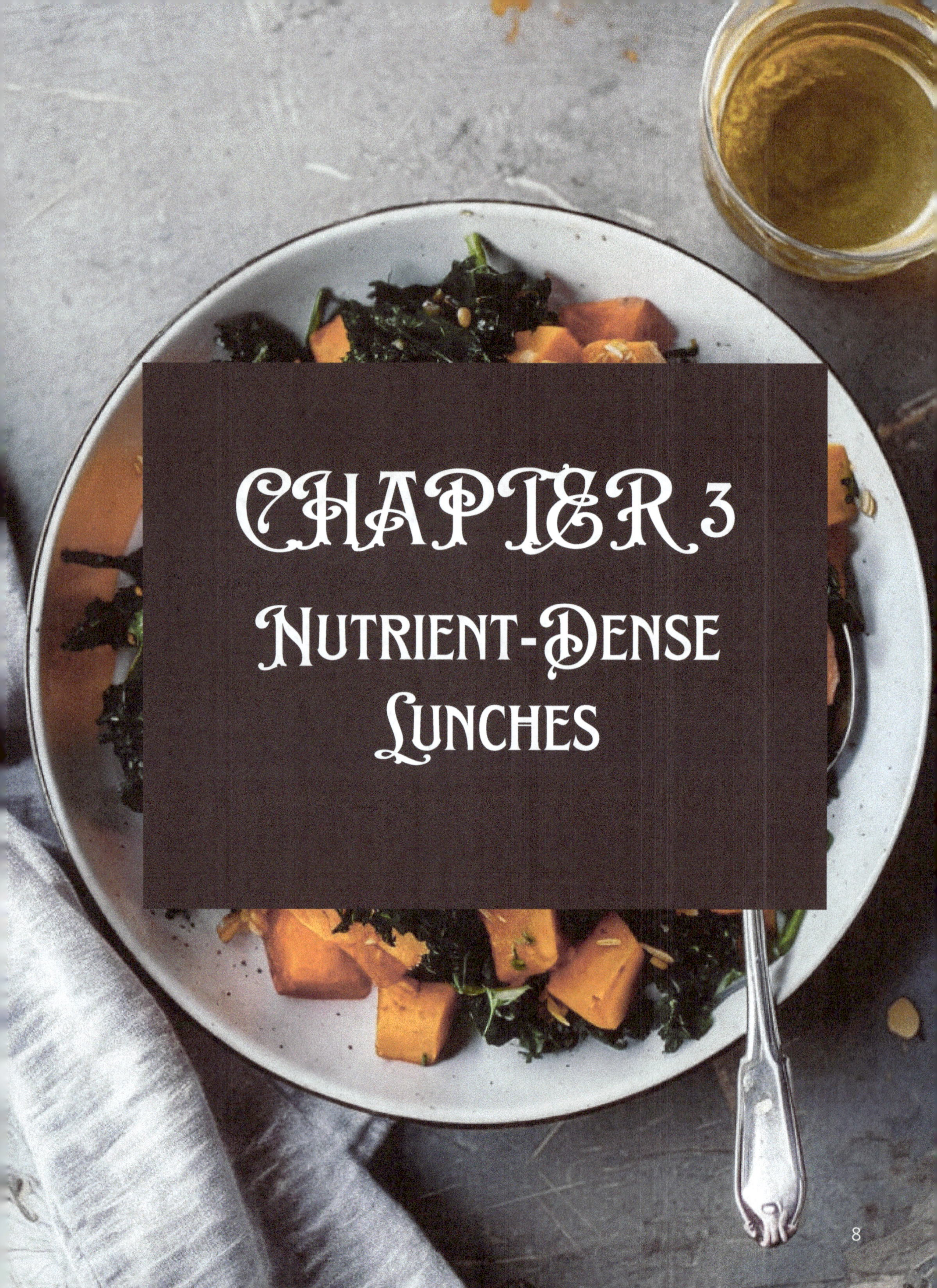

CHAPTER 3
NUTRIENT-DENSE
LUNCHES

SPINACH AND STRAWBERRY SALAD

Ingredients

- 6 cups fresh baby spinach leaves
- 1 pint strawberries, hulled and sliced
- 1/4 cup sliced almonds
- 1/4 cup crumbled feta cheese
- Balsamic vinaigrette dressing

Instructions

- Wash the spinach leaves thoroughly and pat them dry with paper towels or a clean kitchen towel.
- In a large salad bowl, combine the spinach leaves, sliced strawberries, sliced almonds, and crumbled feta cheese.
- Drizzle the desired amount of balsamic vinaigrette dressing over the salad. Toss gently to coat all the ingredients evenly.
- Serve immediately as a refreshing side salad or light meal.

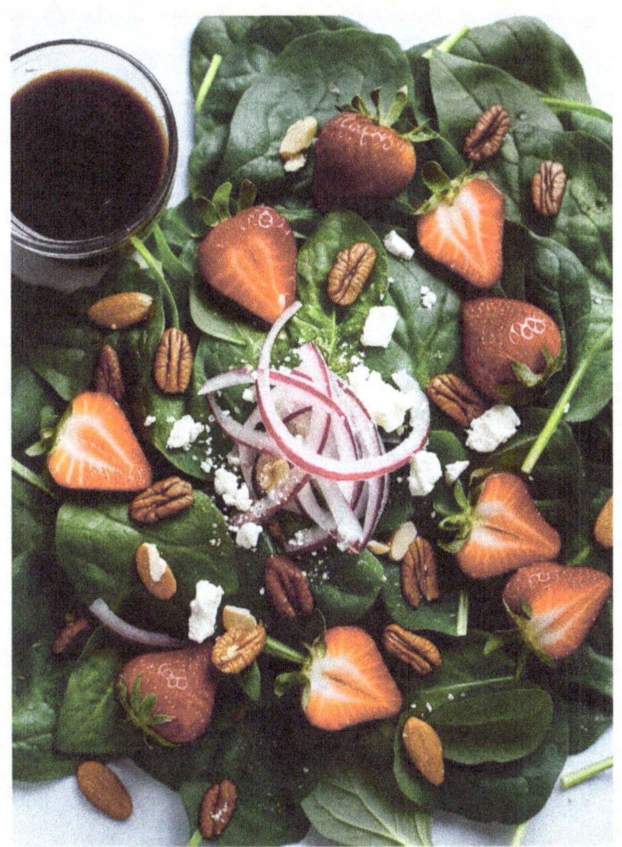

Preparation Time : 10 min

Total Time : 10 min

Servings : 4

Nutritional Info

- Calories: 120
- Total Fat: 7g
- Saturated Fat: 1.5g
- Cholesterol: 5mg
- Sodium: 140mg
- Dietary Fiber: 4g

GRILLED CHICKEN AND VEGETABLE SALAD

Ingredients

- 2 boneless, skinless chicken breasts
- 2 tablespoons olive oil
- 1 teaspoon garlic powder
- Salt and pepper to taste
- 4 cups mixed salad greens
- 1 bell pepper, sliced
- 1 cup cherry tomatoes, halved
- 1 small red onion, thinly sliced
- 1/4 cup balsamic vinaigrette dressing

Instructions

- Preheat your grill to medium-high heat.
- In a small bowl, mix together olive oil, garlic powder, salt, and pepper. Brush this mixture onto both sides of the chicken breasts.
- Grill the chicken breasts for about 6-8 minutes per side, or until cooked through and no longer pink in the center. Remove from the grill and let them rest for a few minutes before slicing.
- While the chicken is cooking, prepare the vegetables. In a large bowl, toss together the mixed salad greens, bell pepper slices, cherry tomatoes, and red onion slices.
- Once the chicken has rested, slice it thinly.
- Arrange the grilled chicken slices on top of the salad vegetables.
- Drizzle the balsamic vinaigrette dressing over the salad.
- Serve immediately and enjoy!

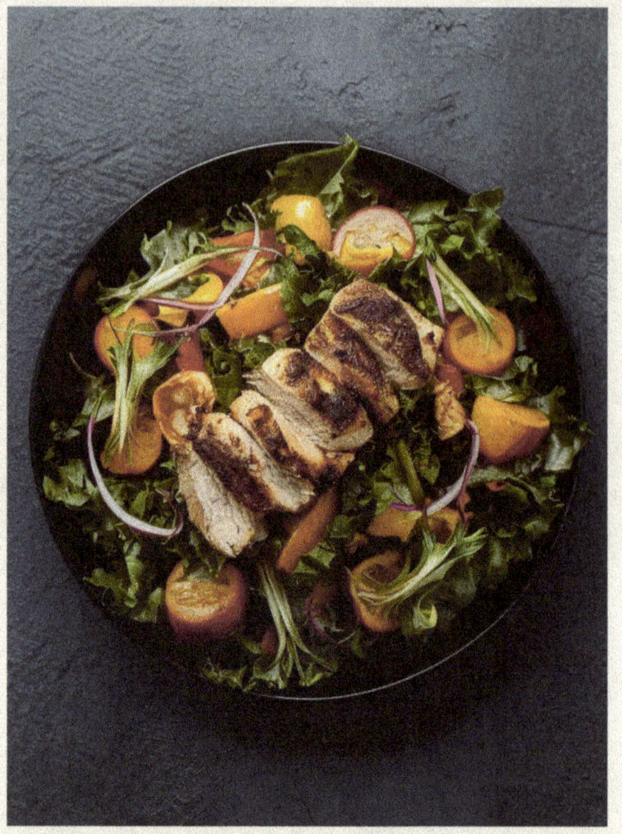

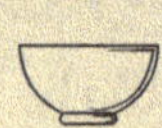 **Preparation Time : 15 min**

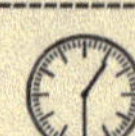 **Total Time : 30 min**

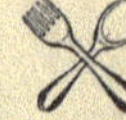 **Servings : 4**

Nutritional Info

- Calories: 250 kcal
- Protein: 25g
- Carbohydrates: 15g
- Fat: 10g
- Fiber: 5g

AVOCADO AND BLACK BEAN WRAP

Ingredients

- 1 can (15 oz) black beans, drained and rinsed
- 1 ripe avocado, diced
- 1 cup cherry tomatoes, halved
- 1/4 cup red onion, finely chopped
- 1/4 cup fresh cilantro, chopped
- Juice of 1 lime
- Salt and pepper to taste
- 4 whole wheat tortillas
- 1/2 cup shredded lettuce (optional)

Instructions

- In a medium bowl, combine black beans, avocado, cherry tomatoes, red onion, cilantro, lime juice, salt, and pepper. Gently toss to mix all ingredients well.
- Lay the tortillas flat on a clean surface. Divide the black bean and avocado mixture evenly among the tortillas, placing it in the center of each.
- If using, sprinkle shredded lettuce over the mixture.
- Fold the sides of the tortillas over the filling, then roll them up tightly.
- Serve immediately, or wrap in foil or parchment paper to take on the go.

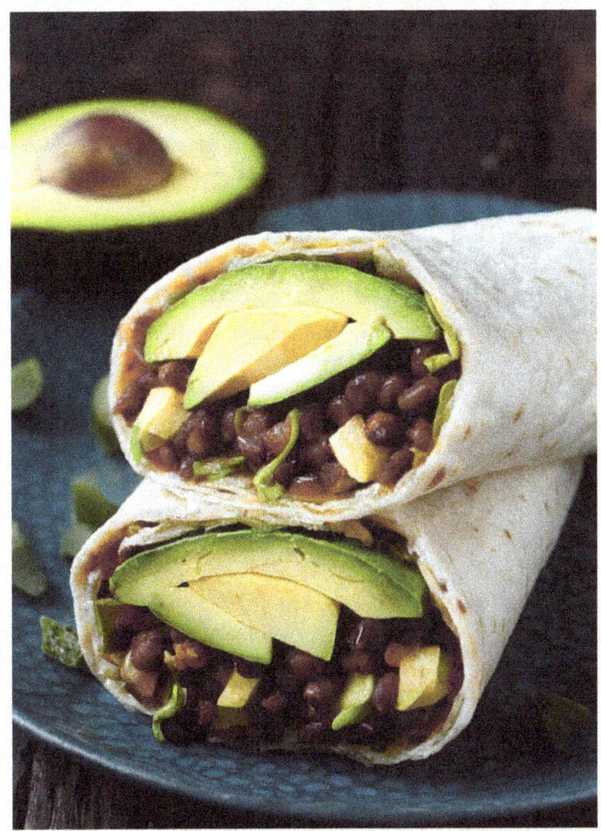

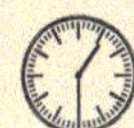 **Preparation Time : 10 min**

 **Total Time : 10 min**

Servings : 4

Nutritional Info

- Calories: 290
- Protein: 10g
- Fat: 10g
- Carbohydrates: 40g
- Fiber: 12g

ROASTED BEET AND GOAT CHEESE SALAD

Ingredients

- 4 medium beets, washed and trimmed
- 2 tablespoons olive oil
- Salt and pepper to taste
- 4 cups mixed greens (e.g., arugula, spinach, and kale)
- 1/2 cup crumbled goat cheese
- 1/4 cup chopped walnuts
- 1/4 cup balsamic vinaigrette

Instructions

- Preheat your oven to 400°F (200°C).
- Wrap each beet in aluminum foil and place them on a baking sheet.
- Roast for 45 minutes or until tender when pierced with a fork.
- Remove from the oven and let cool.
- Once cooled, peel the beets and cut them into wedges.
- In a large bowl, toss the mixed greens with olive oil, salt, and pepper.
- Add the roasted beet wedges, crumbled goat cheese, and chopped walnuts.
- Drizzle the balsamic vinaigrette over the salad and gently toss to combine.
- Divide the salad among four plates and serve immediately.

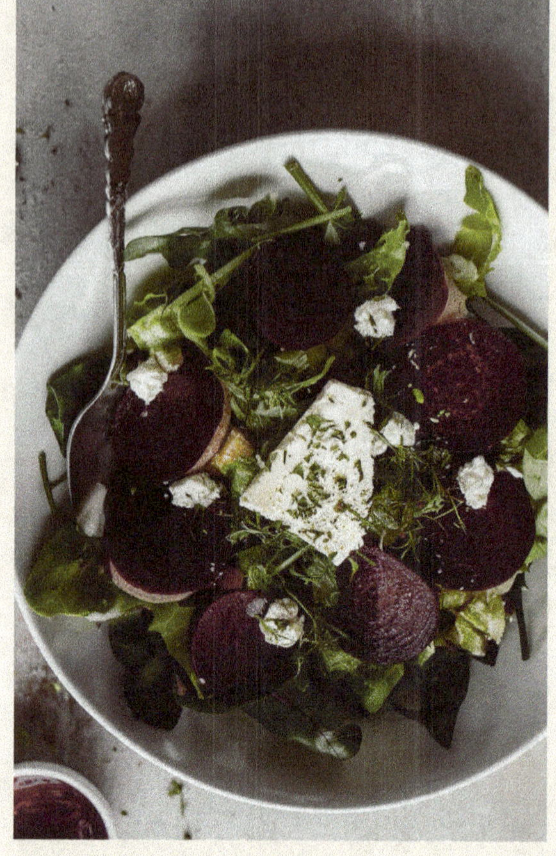

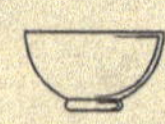 **Preparation Time : 15 min**

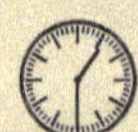 **Total Time : 60 min**

 **Servings : 4**

Nutritional Info

- Calories: 210
- Protein: 6g
- Carbohydrates: 18g
- Fat: 14g
- Fiber: 4g

SALMON AND ASPARAGUS SALAD

Ingredients

- 2 salmon fillets
- 1 bunch of asparagus, trimmed
- 2 tablespoons olive oil
- Salt and pepper to taste
- 4 cups mixed salad greens
- 1 avocado, sliced
- 1/4 cup cherry tomatoes, halved
- 2 tablespoons balsamic vinegar

Instructions

- Preheat oven to 400°F (200°C).
- Place salmon fillets on a baking sheet lined with parchment paper. Drizzle with 1 tablespoon of olive oil and season with salt and pepper. Bake for 12-15 minutes until salmon is cooked through.
- While the salmon is baking, toss asparagus spears with the remaining olive oil, salt, and pepper. Roast in the oven for 8-10 minutes until tender but still crisp.
- In a large bowl, combine mixed salad greens, avocado slices, and cherry tomatoes.
- Once the salmon and asparagus are cooked, let them cool slightly. Then, flake the salmon into chunks and add it to the salad along with the asparagus.
- Drizzle balsamic vinegar over the salad and gently toss to combine.
- Serve immediately.

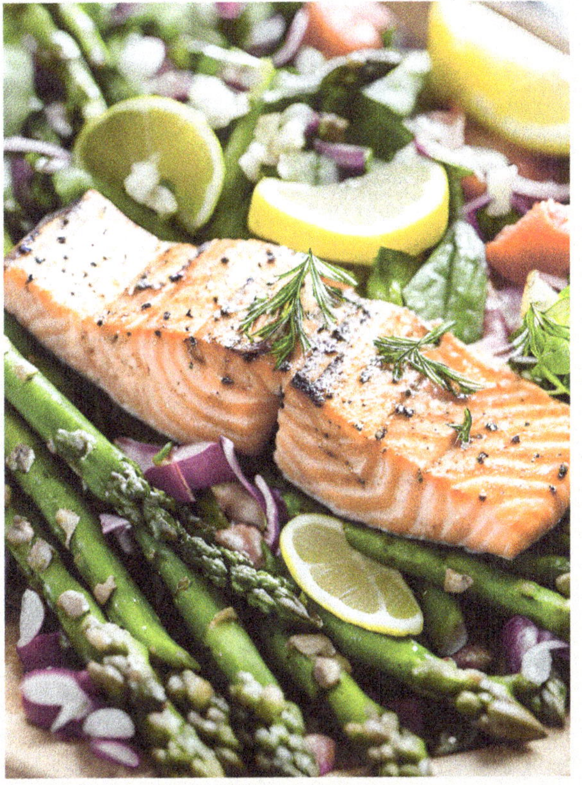

Preparation Time : 10 min

Total Time : 25 min

Servings : 2

Nutritional Info

- Calories: 450 kcal
- Protein: 28g
- Carbohydrates: 15g
- Fat: 33g
- Fiber: 9g

SWEET POTATO AND LENTIL STEW

Ingredients

- 1 tablespoon olive oil
- 1 onion, chopped
- 2 cloves garlic, minced
- 2 medium sweet potatoes, peeled and diced
- 1 cup dried green lentils, rinsed
- 4 cups vegetable broth
- 1 can (14 ounces) diced tomatoes
- 1 teaspoon ground cumin
- 1 teaspoon ground coriander
- Salt and pepper to taste

Instructions

- In a large pot or Dutch oven, heat the olive oil over medium heat.
- Add the chopped onion and minced garlic. Sauté until the onion is translucent, about 3-4 minutes.
- Add the diced sweet potatoes and rinsed lentils to the pot.
- Pour in the vegetable broth and diced tomatoes. Stir to combine.
- Season the stew with ground cumin, ground coriander, salt, and pepper.
- Bring the stew to a simmer, then reduce the heat to low. Cover and cook for 25-30 minutes, or until the sweet potatoes and lentils are tender.
- Taste and adjust seasoning if needed.
- Serve the stew hot, garnished with fresh cilantro or parsley if desired.

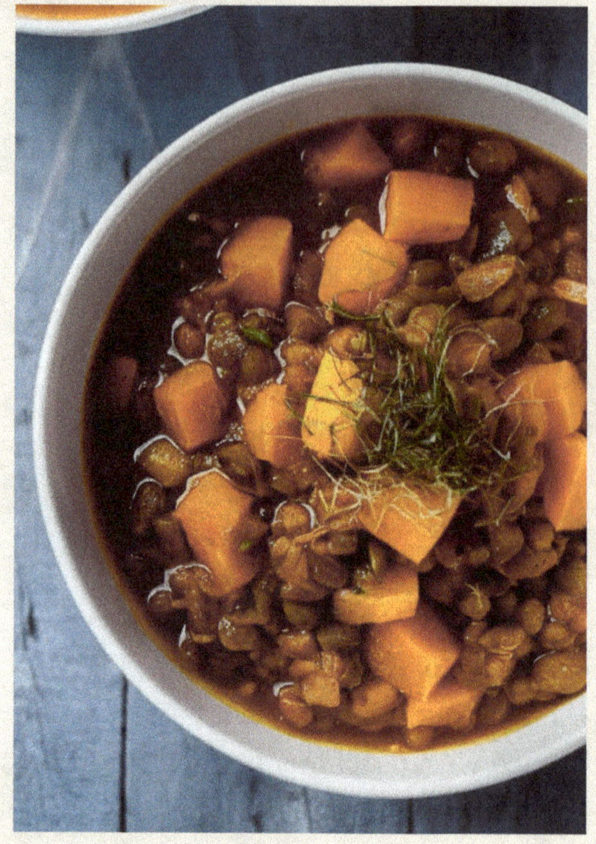

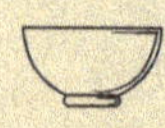 **Preparation Time : 10 min**

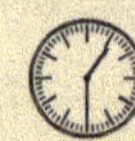 **Total Time : 40 min**

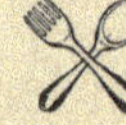 **Servings : 4**

Nutritional Info

- Calories: 315 kcal
- Protein: 13g
- Carbohydrates: 58g
- Fat: 4g
- Fiber: 15g

TOFU AND BROCCOLI STIR-FRY

Ingredients

- 1 block firm tofu, drained and cubed
- 2 cups broccoli florets
- 2 tablespoons soy sauce (or tamari for gluten-free)
- 1 tablespoon sesame oil
- 2 cloves garlic, minced
- 1 tablespoon grated ginger
- 2 tablespoons olive oil (for cooking)

Instructions

- Heat olive oil in a large skillet or wok over medium-high heat.
- Add cubed tofu to the skillet and cook until golden brown on all sides, about 5-7 minutes. Remove tofu from skillet and set aside.
- In the same skillet, add broccoli florets and cook for 3-4 minutes until they are bright green and slightly tender.
- Add minced garlic and grated ginger to the skillet, stirring constantly for about 1 minute until fragrant.
- Return the cooked tofu to the skillet and pour soy sauce and sesame oil over the tofu and broccoli mixture. Stir well to coat everything evenly.
- Cook for an additional 2-3 minutes until the sauce has thickened slightly and everything is heated through.
- Remove from heat and garnish with sesame seeds and sliced green onions if desired.
- Serve hot over cooked rice or quinoa.

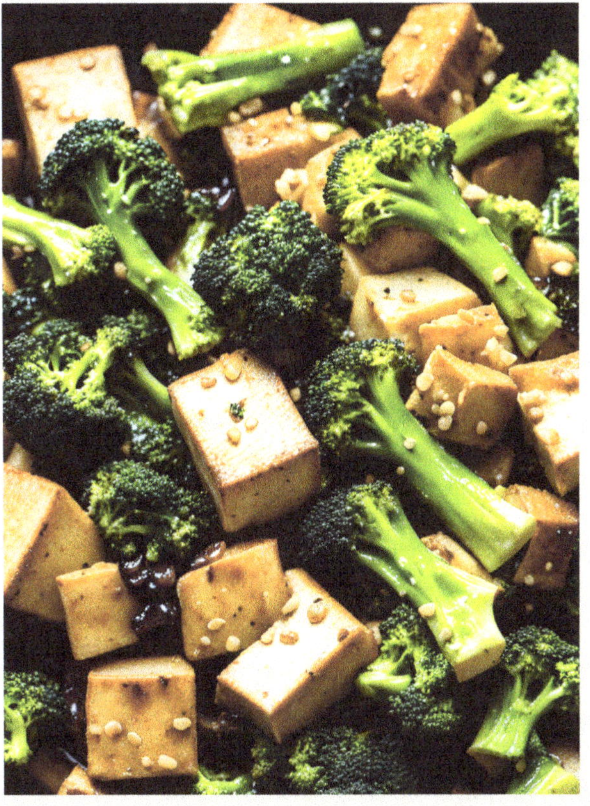

Preparation Time : 10min

Total Time : 20 min

Servings : 2

Nutritional Info

- Calories: 250 kcal
- Protein: 15g
- Carbohydrates: 10g
- Fat: 18g
- Fiber: 5g

SPICY TUNA AND AVOCADO BOWL

Ingredients

- 1 can (5 oz) of tuna in water, drained
- 1 ripe avocado, diced
- 1 cup cooked brown rice (optional, adjust points if included)
- 1 cup mixed greens
- 1/2 cup shredded carrots
- 1/2 cup sliced cucumber
- 1/4 cup chopped green onions
- 1 tbsp soy sauce (low sodium)
- 1 tsp sesame oil
- 1 tsp Sriracha (adjust to taste)
- 1 tbsp lime juice
- 1 tbsp sesame seeds

Instructions

- Prepare the Ingredients: Drain the tuna and place it in a medium bowl. Dice the avocado and set aside. Cook the brown rice if using.
- Make the Dressing: In a small bowl, whisk together the soy sauce, sesame oil, Sriracha, and lime juice.
- Combine Ingredients: In the bowl with the tuna, add the mixed greens, shredded carrots, sliced cucumber, chopped green onions, and diced avocado. Pour the dressing over the mixture.
- Mix Well: Gently toss all the ingredients together until evenly coated with the dressing.
- Serve: Divide the mixture into bowls, sprinkle with sesame seeds, and season with salt and pepper to taste. Serve immediately.
- Optional: Serve over a bed of cooked brown rice for a heartier meal.

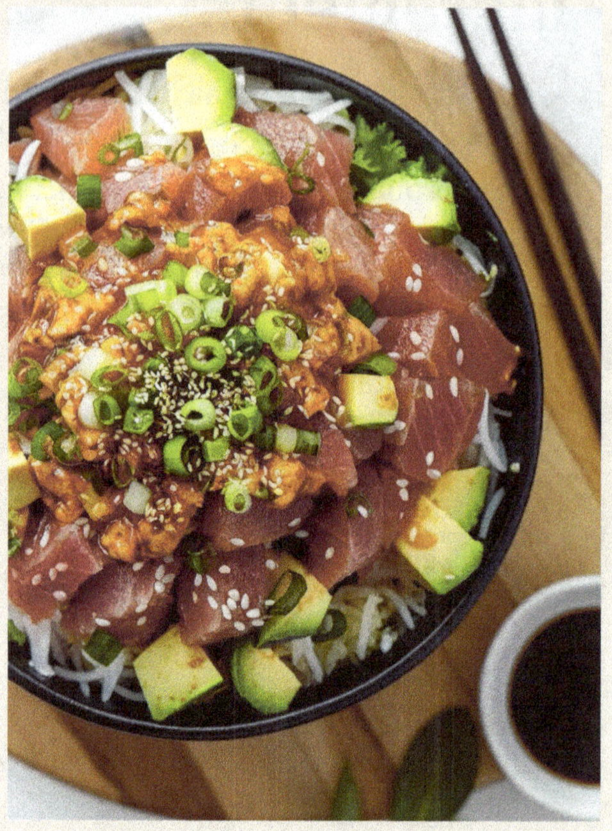

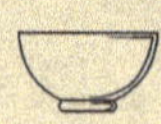 **Preparation Time : 10 min**

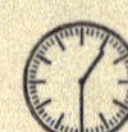 **Total Time : 10 min**

 **Servings : 1**

Nutritional Info

- Calories: 320 (without brown rice)
- Protein: 20g
- Carbohydrates: 14g
- Fat: 22g
- Fiber: 8g

CHICKEN CAESAR SALAD

Ingredients

- 2 boneless, skinless chicken breasts
- 1 tablespoon olive oil
- 1 teaspoon garlic powder
- Salt and pepper to taste
- 1 large head of romaine lettuce, chopped
- 1/2 cup cherry tomatoes, halved
- 1/4 cup grated Parmesan cheese
- 1/2 cup croutons (optional)
- Lemon wedges for garnish

Instructions

- Preheat your oven to 375°F (190°C).
- Rub the chicken breasts with olive oil, garlic powder, salt, and pepper.
- Place the chicken breasts on a baking sheet and bake for 20 minutes, or until the internal temperature reaches 165°F (74°C).
- Allow the chicken to rest for 5 minutes before slicing.
- While the chicken is baking, chop the romaine lettuce and place it in a large salad bowl.
- Add the halved cherry tomatoes and grated Parmesan cheese to the bowl.
- If using croutons, add them to the salad as well.
- Once the chicken has rested, slice it into thin strips.
- Arrange the sliced chicken on top of the salad.
- Serve the salad with lemon wedges on the side for squeezing over the top.
- Divide the salad into four servings.
- Enjoy your Chicken Caesar Salad without dressing, optionally squeezing fresh lemon juice over the top for extra flavor.

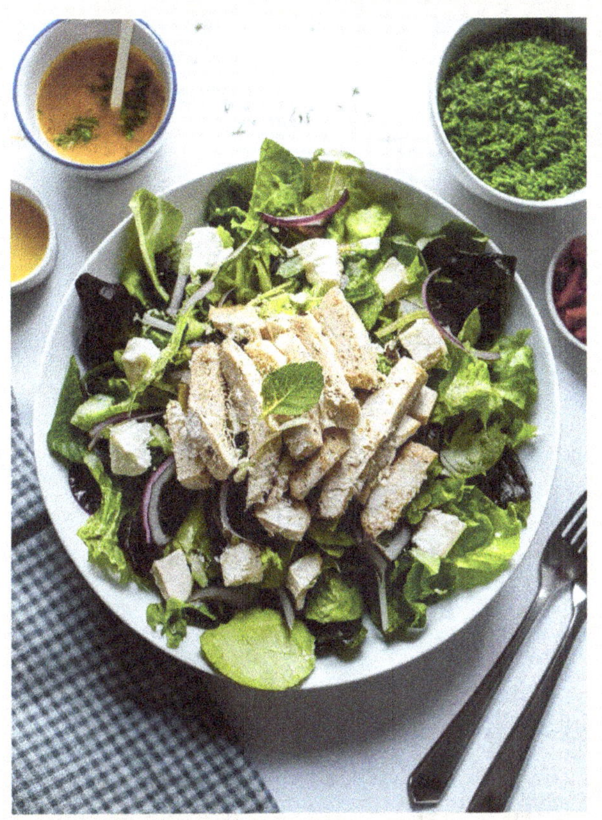

🥣 **Preparation Time : 15 min**

🕐 **Total Time : 35 min**

🍴 **Servings : 4**

Nutritional Info

- Calories: 220
- Protein: 30g
- Carbohydrates: 8g
- Fat: 8g
- Fiber: 2g

MEDITERRANEAN CHICKPEA BOWL

Ingredients

- 1 can (15 oz) chickpeas, drained and rinsed
- 1 cup cherry tomatoes, halved
- 1 cucumber, diced
- 1/2 red onion, thinly sliced
- 1/4 cup Kalamata olives, pitted and sliced
- 2 tablespoons extra virgin olive oil
- 1 tablespoon lemon juice
- 1 teaspoon dried oregano
- Salt and pepper to taste

Instructions

- In a large bowl, combine the chickpeas, cherry tomatoes, cucumber, red onion, and Kalamata olives.
- In a small bowl, whisk together the extra virgin olive oil, lemon juice, dried oregano, salt, and pepper.
- Pour the dressing over the chickpea mixture and toss until well combined.
- Divide the chickpea mixture into serving bowls.
- Top with crumbled feta cheese and fresh parsley if desired.
- Serve immediately and enjoy!

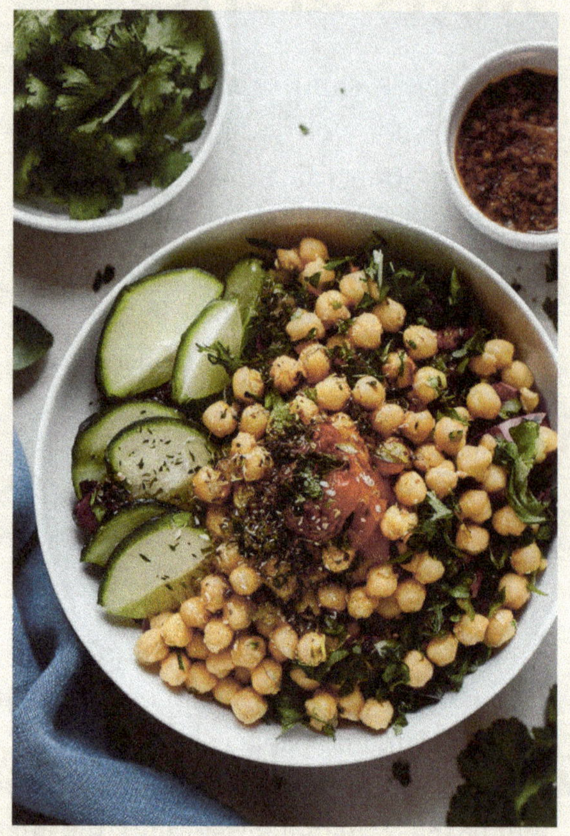

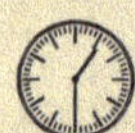 **Preparation Time : 10 min**

 **Total Time : 10 min**

Servings : 2

Nutritional Info

- Calories: 320 kcal
- Total Fat: 18g
- Saturated Fat: 2.5g
- Trans Fat: 0g
- Cholesterol: 0mg

Chapter 4

Healing Dinners

BAKED SALMON WITH LEMON AND DILL

Ingredients

- 4 salmon fillets
- 2 tablespoons olive oil
- 2 tablespoons fresh lemon juice
- 2 cloves garlic, minced
- 1 tablespoon fresh dill, chopped
- Salt and pepper, to taste
- Lemon slices, for garnish

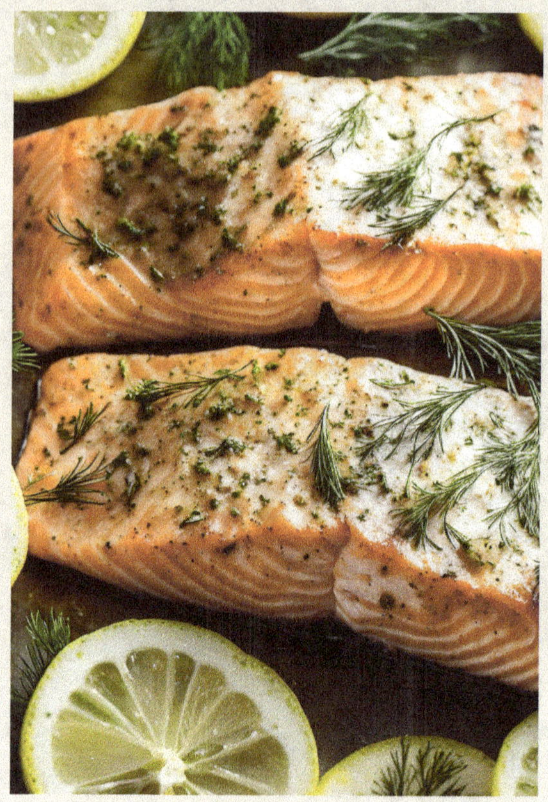

Instructions

- Preheat your oven to 375°F (190°C). Line a baking sheet with parchment paper or lightly grease it with olive oil.
- In a small bowl, mix together the olive oil, lemon juice, minced garlic, chopped dill, salt, and pepper.
- Place the salmon fillets on the prepared baking sheet. Brush each fillet with the lemon-dill mixture, coating them evenly.
- Place a lemon slice on top of each salmon fillet for added flavor.
- Bake the salmon in the preheated oven for 12-15 minutes, or until the salmon is cooked through and flakes easily with a fork.
- Once done, remove the salmon from the oven and garnish with fresh dill sprigs.
- Serve the baked salmon hot with your favorite side dishes.

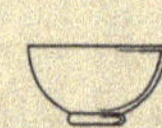 **Preparation Time : 10 min**

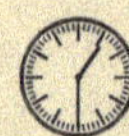 **Total Time : 20 min**

 **Servings : 4**

Nutritional Info

- Calories: 280 kcal
- Protein: 25g
- Fat: 18g
- Carbohydrates: 2g
- Fiber: 0.5g

QUINOA AND VEGETABLE STUFFED PEPPERS

Ingredients

- 4 large bell peppers, any color
- 1 cup quinoa, rinsed
- 2 cups vegetable broth
- 1 tablespoon olive oil
- 1 onion, diced
- 2 cloves garlic, minced
- 1 zucchini, diced
- 1 carrot, diced
- 1 cup diced tomatoes
- 1 teaspoon dried oregano
- Salt and pepper to taste

Instructions

- Preheat oven to 375°F (190°C).
- Cook quinoa: In a saucepan, combine quinoa and vegetable broth. Bring to a boil, then simmer covered for 15 minutes until cooked.
- Prepare vegetables: Heat olive oil in a skillet. Add onion and garlic, cook until softened (about 5 mins). Then add zucchini and carrot, cook for another 5 mins until tender.
- Mix: Stir in diced tomatoes, oregano, cooked quinoa, salt, and pepper. Cook for 2-3 more minutes.
- Prepare peppers: Cut the tops off the bell peppers, remove seeds and membranes. Place in a baking dish.
- Fill peppers: Spoon quinoa and vegetable mixture into each pepper.
- Optional: Sprinkle shredded mozzarella cheese on top.
- Bake: Cover dish with foil, bake for 25-30 mins until peppers are tender.
- Serve hot and enjoy!

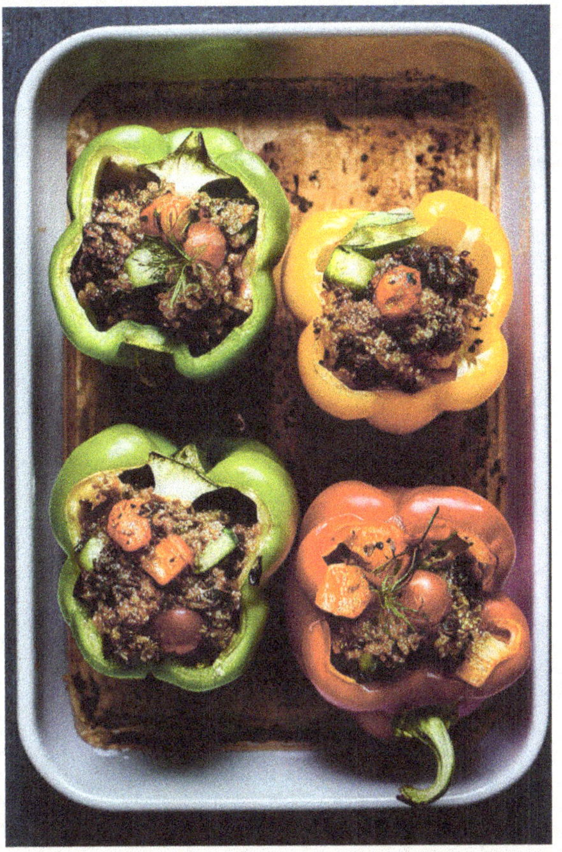

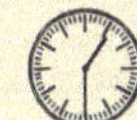 **Preparation Time : 20 min**

 **Total Time : 1 hour**

Servings : 4

Nutritional Info

- Calories: 295 kcal
- Total Fat: 7g
- Saturated Fat: 1g
- Cholesterol: 0mg
- Sodium: 460mg

Ingredients

- 1 lb boneless, skinless chicken breasts, cut into bite-sized pieces
- 2 cups white or brown rice
- 1 tablespoon olive oil
- 1 onion, chopped
- 3 cloves garlic, minced
- 1 tablespoon ground turmeric
- 1 teaspoon ground cumin
- 1 teaspoon ground coriander
- Salt and pepper to taste
- 3 cups chicken broth
- 1 cup frozen peas

Instructions

- Heat olive oil in a large skillet over medium heat. Add chopped onion and minced garlic, sauté until softened.
- Add chicken pieces to the skillet, cook until browned on all sides.
- Stir in ground turmeric, cumin, and coriander, coating the chicken evenly.
- Add rice to the skillet, stirring to combine with the chicken and spices.
- Pour chicken broth into the skillet, bring to a boil.
- Reduce heat to low, cover, and simmer for 20-25 minutes or until rice is cooked and liquid is absorbed.
- Stir in frozen peas, cover, and cook for an additional 5 minutes until peas are heated through.
- Garnish with chopped cilantro before serving.

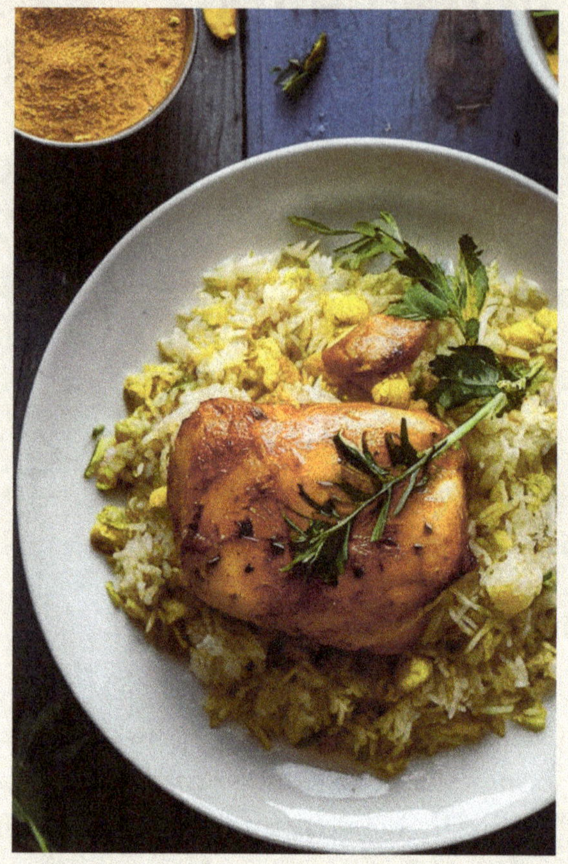

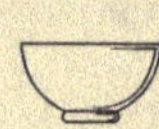 **Preparation Time : 10 min**

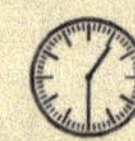 **Total Time : 35 min**

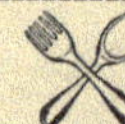 **Servings : 4**

Nutritional Info

- Calories: 400 kcal
- Protein: 30g
- Carbohydrates: 45g
- Fat: 10g
- Fiber: 4g

SWEET POTATO AND BLACK BEAN ENCHILADAS

Ingredients

- 2 medium sweet potatoes, peeled and diced
- 1 can (15 oz) black beans, drained and rinsed
- 1 cup corn kernels (fresh or frozen)
- 1 bell pepper, diced
- 1 small onion, diced
- 2 cloves garlic, minced
- 1 teaspoon ground cumin
- 1 teaspoon chili powder
- Salt and pepper, to taste
- 8 small corn tortillas
- 1 cup enchilada sauce
- 1 cup shredded cheese

Instructions

- Preheat oven to 375°F (190°C). Grease a baking dish.
- In a skillet over medium heat, cook sweet potatoes until soft, about 5-7 minutes.
- Add onion, bell pepper, and garlic. Cook until tender, about 5 minutes.
- Stir in black beans, corn, cumin, chili powder, salt, and pepper. Cook for 2-3 minutes.
- Warm tortillas in the microwave for 30 seconds.
- Spoon filling onto each tortilla. Roll up and place seam-side down in the baking dish.
- Pour enchilada sauce over the top. Sprinkle cheese evenly.
- Cover with foil and bake for 20 minutes.
- Remove foil and bake for 5-10 more minutes, until cheese melts.
- Garnish with cilantro if desired before serving.

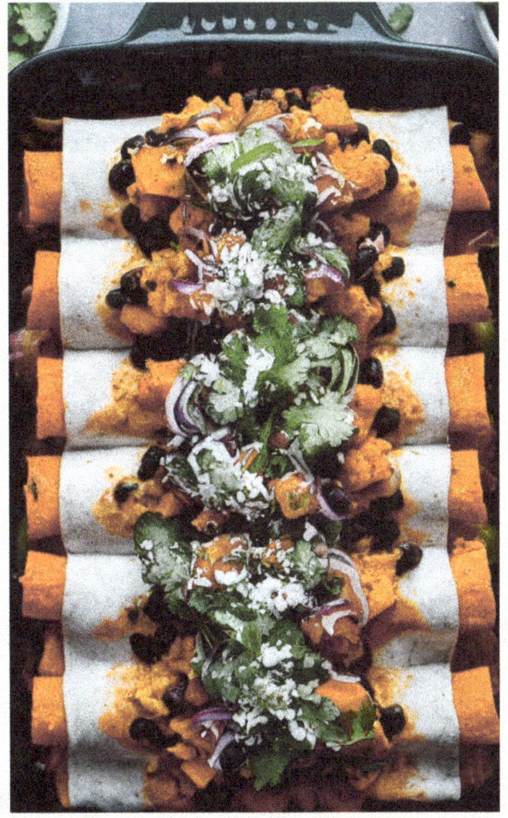

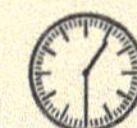 **Preparation Time : 15 min**

 **Total Time : 35 min**

Servings : 4

Nutritional Info

- Calories: 380
- Total Fat: 10g
- Saturated Fat: 5g
- Cholesterol: 20mg
- Sodium: 680mg
- Total Carbohydrates: 59g

Ingredients

- 4 medium zucchinis, spiralized
- 1 cup fresh basil leaves
- 1/4 cup pine nuts
- 2 cloves garlic
- 1/4 cup grated Parmesan cheese
- 1/4 cup olive oil
- Salt and pepper to taste

Instructions

- In a food processor, combine basil leaves, pine nuts, garlic, and Parmesan cheese. Pulse until finely chopped.
- With the processor running, slowly drizzle in the olive oil until the mixture forms a smooth paste. Season with salt and pepper to taste.
- In a large skillet over medium heat, add the spiralized zucchini noodles. Cook for 2-3 minutes until slightly softened but still crisp.
- Add the pesto sauce to the skillet with the zucchini noodles and toss until well coated.
- Serve immediately, garnished with sliced cherry tomatoes if desired.

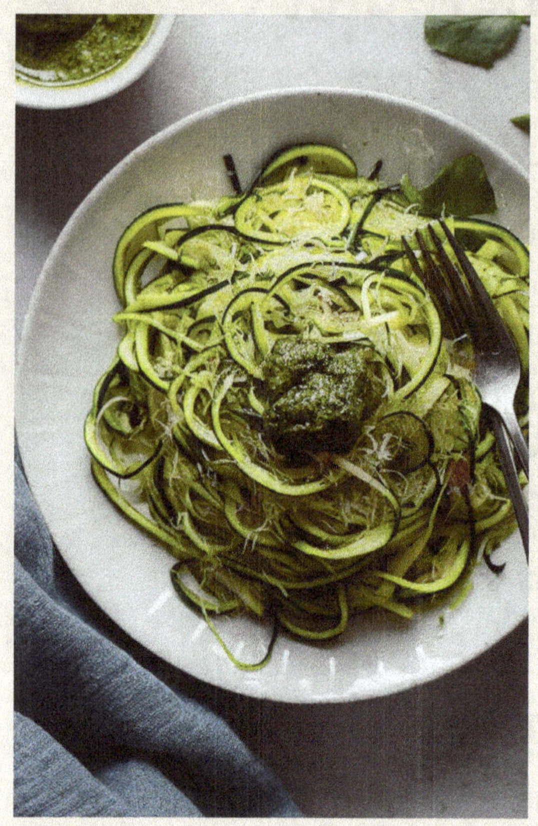

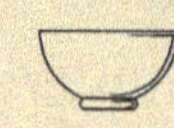
Preparation Time : 10 min

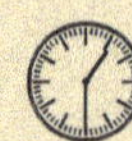
Total Time : 15 min

Servings : 4

Nutritional Info

- Calories: 180 kcal
- Protein: 5g
- Fat: 16g
- Carbohydrates: 7g
- Fiber: 2g

HERB-ROASTED CHICKEN AND VEGETABLES

Ingredients

- 4 bone-in, skin-on chicken thighs
- 2 cups baby potatoes, halved
- 2 cups carrots, peeled and sliced into sticks
- 1 cup Brussels sprouts, halved
- 2 tablespoons olive oil
- 2 cloves garlic, minced
- 1 teaspoon dried thyme
- 1 teaspoon dried rosemary
- 1 teaspoon dried oregano
- Salt and pepper to taste

Instructions

- Preheat your oven to 400°F (200°C).
- In a large mixing bowl, combine the chicken thighs, potatoes, carrots, Brussels sprouts, olive oil, minced garlic, dried thyme, dried rosemary, dried oregano, salt, and pepper. Toss until everything is evenly coated.
- Transfer the chicken and vegetable mixture to a baking sheet lined with parchment paper or aluminum foil, arranging everything in a single layer.
- Roast in the preheated oven for 35-40 minutes or until the chicken is cooked through and the vegetables are tender and golden brown.
- Serve hot, garnished with fresh herbs if desired.

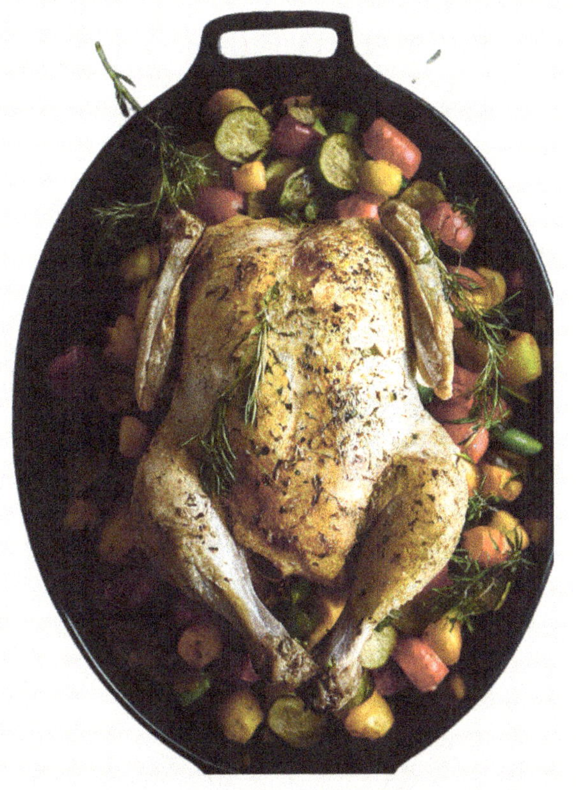

Preparation Time : 15 min

Total Time : 55 min

Servings : 4

Nutritional Info

- Calories: 380 kcal
- Total Fat: 20g
- Saturated Fat: 5g
- Trans Fat: 0g
- Cholesterol: 120mg
- Sodium: 210mg

GINGER-GARLIC SHRIMP STIR-FRY

Ingredients

- 1 lb shrimp, peeled and deveined
- 2 tablespoons olive oil
- 3 cloves garlic, minced
- 1 tablespoon fresh ginger, minced
- 1 red bell pepper, thinly sliced
- 1 yellow bell pepper, thinly sliced
- 1 cup snow peas
- 1/4 cup low-sodium soy sauce
- 2 tablespoons honey
- 2 green onions, chopped

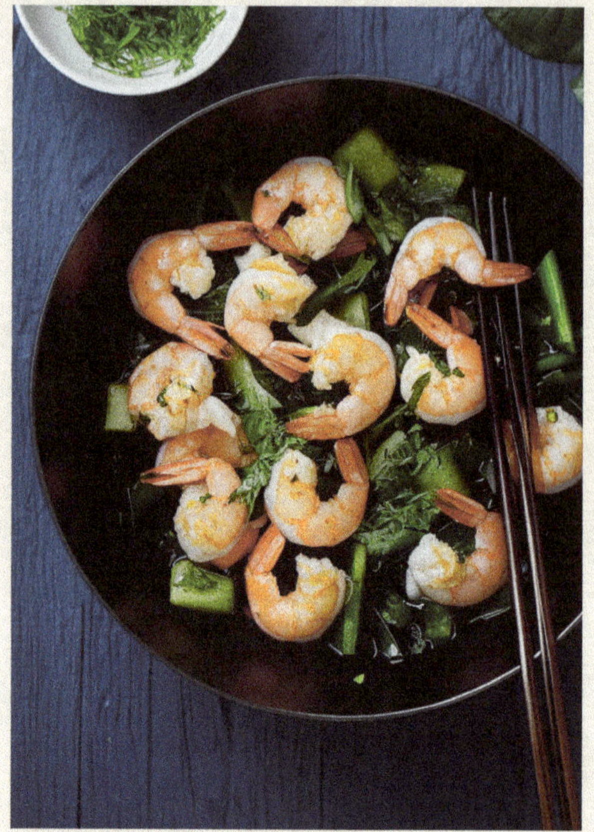

Instructions

- In a large pan, heat olive oil over medium-high heat.
- Add garlic and ginger, sauté for 1-2 minutes until fragrant.
- Add shrimp and cook for 3-4 minutes until pink and cooked through.
- Stir in bell peppers and snow peas, cook for an additional 2-3 minutes.
- In a small bowl, mix soy sauce and honey. Pour over the shrimp and vegetables, stirring to combine.
- Cook for another 1-2 minutes, until the sauce has thickened slightly.
- Remove from heat and sprinkle with chopped green onions.
- Serve over cooked rice.

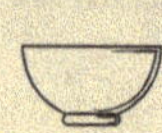 **Preparation Time : 15 min**

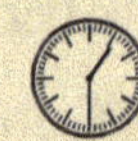 **Total Time : 25 min**

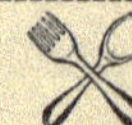 **Servings : 4**

Nutritional Info

- Calories: 280
- Protein: 25g
- Fat: 10g
- Carbohydrates: 20g
- Fiber: 3g

LENTIL AND SPINACH CURRY

Ingredients

- 1 cup dried lentils
- 2 cups fresh spinach, chopped
- 1 onion, finely chopped
- 2 cloves garlic, minced
- 1 tablespoon curry powder
- 1 teaspoon ground cumin
- 1 teaspoon ground coriander
- 1 can (14 ounces) diced tomatoes
- 1 can (14 ounces) coconut milk
- Salt and pepper, to taste

Instructions

- Rinse the lentils under cold water until the water runs clear. Drain well.
- In a large pot or skillet, heat some oil over medium heat. Add the chopped onion and minced garlic, and sauté until softened and fragrant, about 3-4 minutes.
- Stir in the curry powder, ground cumin, and ground coriander. Cook for another minute until the spices are toasted and fragrant.
- Add the rinsed lentils, diced tomatoes (with their juices), and coconut milk to the pot. Stir to combine.
- Bring the mixture to a boil, then reduce the heat to low. Cover and simmer for about 20-25 minutes, or until the lentils are tender and cooked through.
- Stir in the chopped spinach and cook for an additional 2-3 minutes, until the spinach is wilted.
- Season with salt and pepper to taste.
- Serve the lentil and spinach curry hot over cooked rice. Garnish with fresh cilantro.

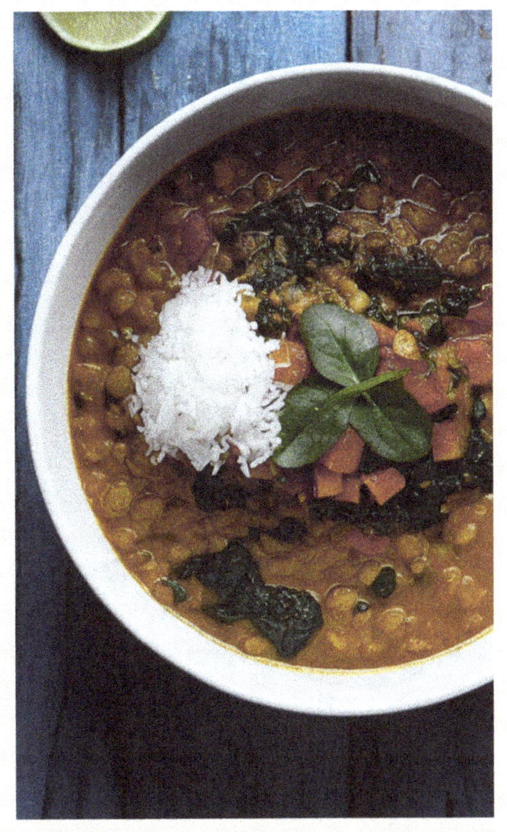

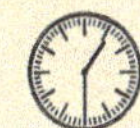 **Preparation Time : 10 min**

 **Total Time : 35 min**

Servings : 4

Nutritional Info

- Calories: 320 kcal
- Protein: 15g
- Carbohydrates: 40g
- Fat: 12g
- Fiber: 14g

ROASTED CAULIFLOWER STEAKS

Ingredients

- 1 large head of cauliflower
- 2-3 tablespoons olive oil
- Salt and pepper to taste
- Optional: your favorite seasoning blend (such as garlic powder, smoked paprika, or cumin)

Instructions

- Preheat your oven to 425°F (220°C).
- Remove the outer leaves of the cauliflower and trim the stem end to create a flat base.
- Place the cauliflower head on a cutting board and slice it vertically into 1-inch thick slices, creating "steaks." You should get 2-3 steaks from one head of cauliflower.
- Place the cauliflower steaks on a baking sheet lined with parchment paper or aluminum foil.
- Drizzle olive oil over the cauliflower steaks and use your hands to rub it evenly on both sides.
- Season the cauliflower steaks with salt, pepper, and any optional seasoning blend of your choice.
- Roast in the preheated oven for 25-30 minutes, flipping halfway through, until the cauliflower is tender and golden brown on the edges.

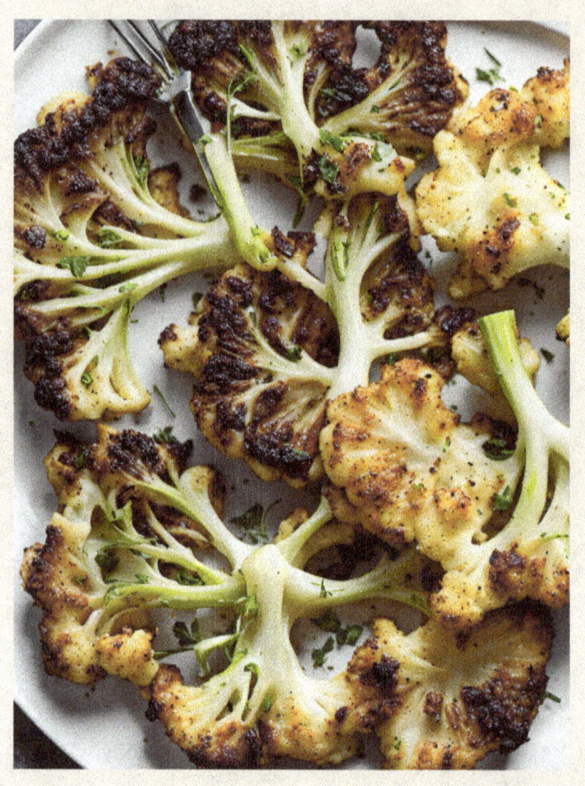

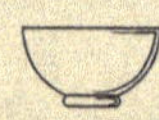 **Preparation Time : 10 min**

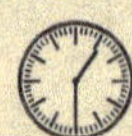 **Total Time : 35 min**

 **Servings : 2-3**

Nutritional Info

- Calories: 120 kcal
- Protein: 5g
- Fat: 9g
- Carbohydrates: 10g
- Fiber: 5g

BAKED COD WITH TOMATO AND OLIVE RELISH

Ingredients

- 4 cod fillets (about 6 oz each)
- 1 cup cherry tomatoes, halved
- 1/4 cup Kalamata olives, chopped
- 2 tablespoons olive oil
- 2 cloves garlic, minced
- 1 tablespoon fresh lemon juice
- Salt and pepper to taste
- Fresh parsley, chopped (for garnish)

Instructions

- Preheat the oven to 400°F (200°C).
- Place the cod fillets on a baking dish lined with parchment paper.
- In a small bowl, mix the cherry tomatoes, olives, olive oil, garlic, lemon juice, salt, and pepper.
- Spoon the tomato and olive mixture over the cod fillets.
- Bake for 15-20 minutes, or until the fish is cooked through and flakes easily with a fork.
- Garnish with fresh parsley before serving.

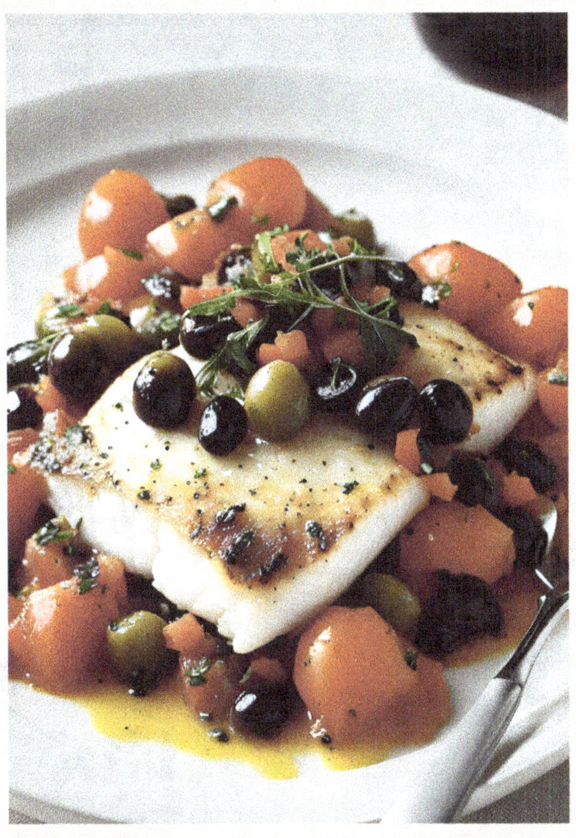

 **Preparation Time : 10 min**

Total Time : 25 min

Servings : 4

Nutritional Info

- Calories: 300
- Protein: 30g
- Fat: 14g
- Carbohydrates: 8g
- Fiber: 2g

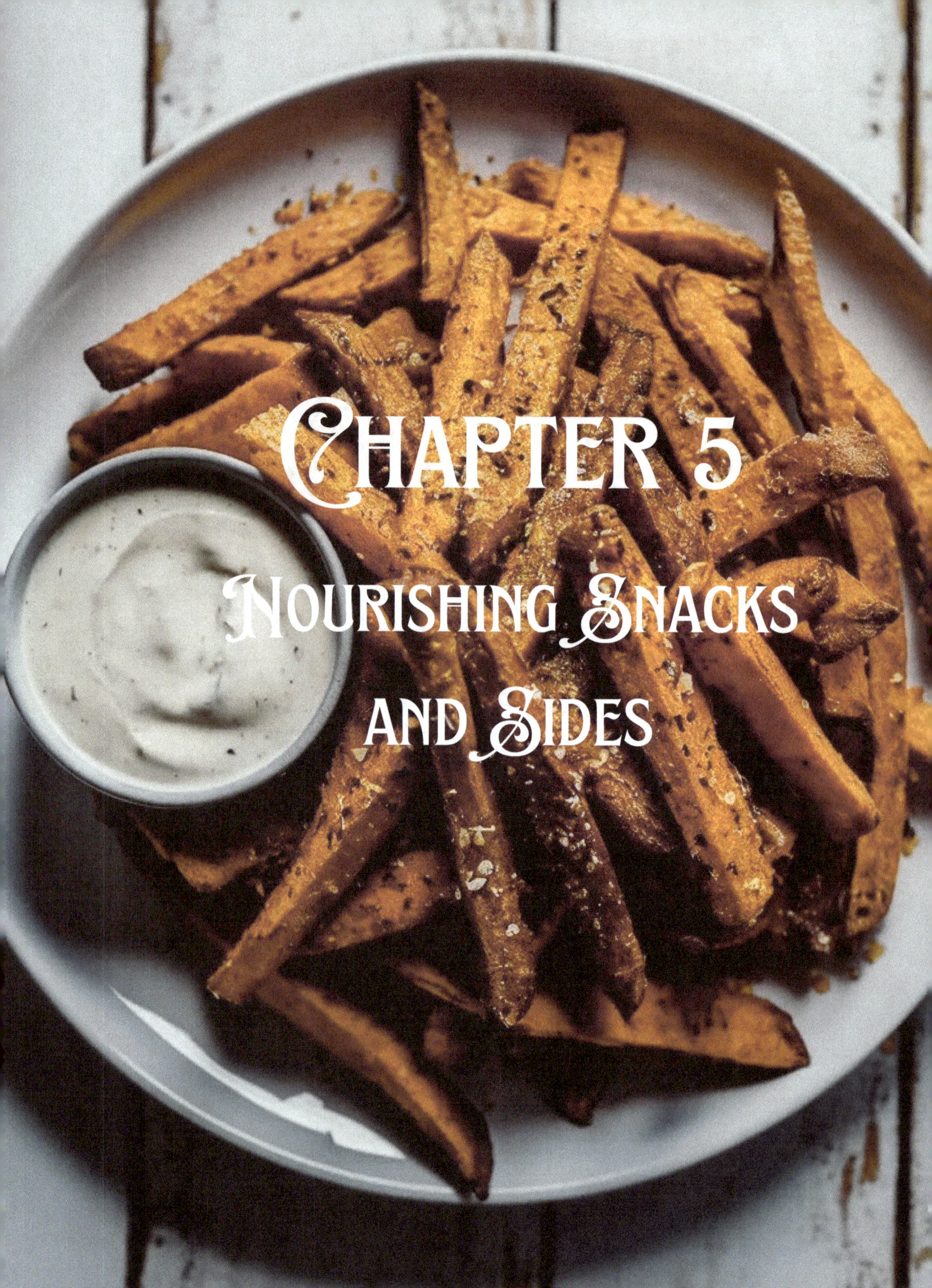
Chapter 5
Nourishing Snacks and Sides

EDAMAME WITH SEA SALT

Ingredients

- 2 cups frozen edamame in pods
- 1 tablespoon sea salt (or to taste)
- Water for boiling

Instructions

- Fill a large pot with water and bring it to a boil over high heat.
- Once the water is boiling, add the frozen edamame pods to the pot.
- Boil for 5 minutes, or until the edamame pods are tender and easily open when squeezed.
- Drain the edamame in a colander and rinse under cold water to stop the cooking process.
- Transfer the edamame to a bowl and sprinkle with sea salt. Toss to evenly coat the pods with the salt.
- Serve immediately as a snack or appetizer.
- To eat, simply squeeze the edamame beans out of the pods and discard the pods.

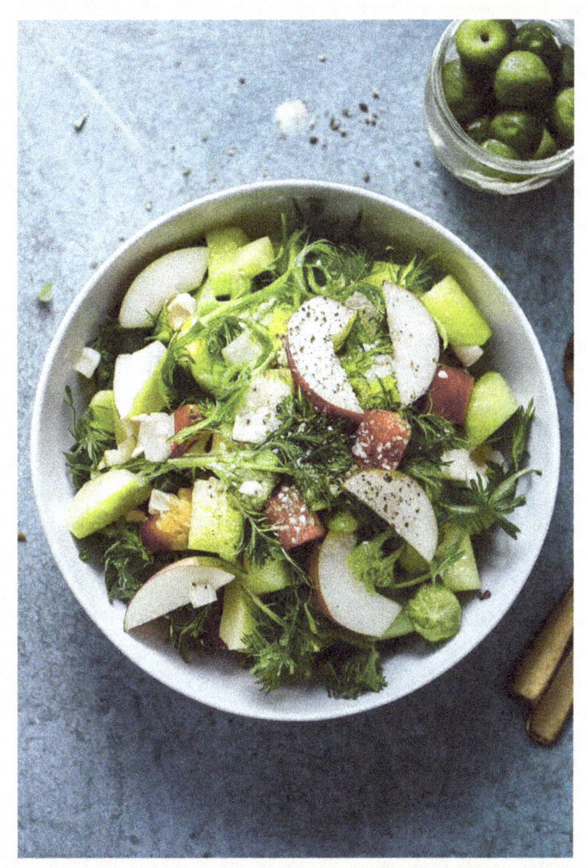

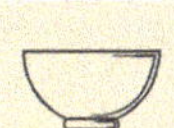 **Preparation Time : 5 min**

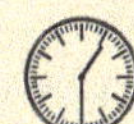 **Total Time : 15 min**

 **Servings : 4**

Nutritional Info

- Calories: 120
- Protein: 12g
- Carbohydrates: 10g
- Fat: 5g
- Fiber: 4g
- Sodium: 150mg

SPICED SWEET POTATO FRIES

Ingredients

- 2 large sweet potatoes
- 1 teaspoon paprika
- 1/2 teaspoon garlic powder
- 1/2 teaspoon onion powder
- 1/2 teaspoon ground cumin
- 1/4 teaspoon cayenne pepper (optional)
- Salt and pepper to taste

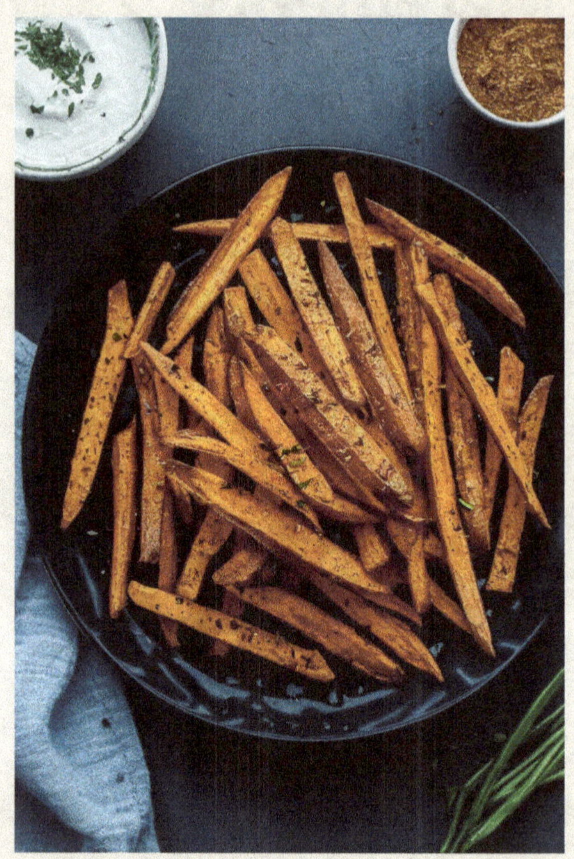

Instructions

- Preheat Oven: Preheat oven to 425°F (220°C). Line a baking sheet with parchment paper or spray with cooking spray.
- Cut Sweet Potatoes: Peel and cut sweet potatoes into thin fries.
- Season: Mix paprika, garlic powder, onion powder, cumin, cayenne pepper (if using), salt, and pepper in a large bowl. Add sweet potatoes and toss to coat.
- Bake: Spread fries on the baking sheet in a single layer. Bake for 20-25 minutes, turning halfway through, until golden and crispy.
- Serve: Let cool slightly and enjoy!

 **Preparation Time : 10 min**

Total Time : 35 min

Servings : 4

Nutritional Info

- Calories: 120
- Protein: 2g
- Carbohydrates: 27g
- Fiber: 4g
- Fat: 0.5g

GUACAMOLE WITH VEGGIE STICKS

Ingredients

- 2 ripe avocados
- 1 small tomato, diced
- 1/4 cup red onion, finely chopped
- 1 jalapeño pepper, seeded and minced (optional for spice)
- 2 tablespoons fresh cilantro, chopped
- 1 tablespoon lime juice
- Salt and pepper to taste

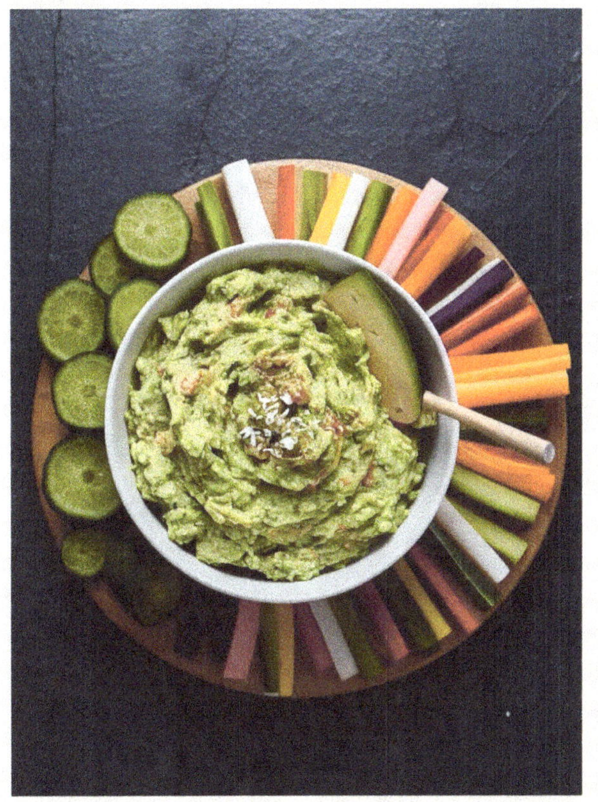

Instructions

- Cut the avocados in half, remove the pits, and scoop the flesh into a mixing bowl.
- Mash the avocados with a fork until smooth or until your desired consistency is reached.
- Add the diced tomato, chopped red onion, minced jalapeño pepper (if using), chopped cilantro, and lime juice to the bowl with the mashed avocado.
- Season with salt and pepper to taste.
- Stir all the ingredients until well combined.
- Taste and adjust seasoning if necessary.
- Transfer the guacamole to a serving bowl and garnish with additional cilantro if desired.
- Serve the guacamole with assorted vegetable sticks for dipping.

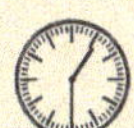 **Preparation Time : 10 min**

 **Total Time : 10 min**

Servings : 4

Nutritional Info

- Calories: 120
- Total Fat: 10g
- Saturated Fat: 1.5g
- Sodium: 250mg
- Total Carbohydrates: 8g
- Dietary Fiber: 6g

ROASTED CHICKPEAS

Ingredients

- 1 can (15 oz) chickpeas, drained and rinsed
- 1 tablespoon olive oil
- 1 teaspoon paprika
- 1 teaspoon garlic powder
- 1/2 teaspoon salt
- 1/4 teaspoon black pepper

Instructions

- Preheat Oven: Preheat your oven to 400°F (200°C).
- Dry Chickpeas: Pat the chickpeas dry with paper towels.
- Season Chickpeas: In a bowl, mix chickpeas with olive oil, paprika, garlic powder, salt, and pepper.
- Bake: Spread chickpeas on a baking sheet. Bake for 35-40 minutes, shaking the pan halfway through.
- Cool: Let cool for a few minutes before serving.

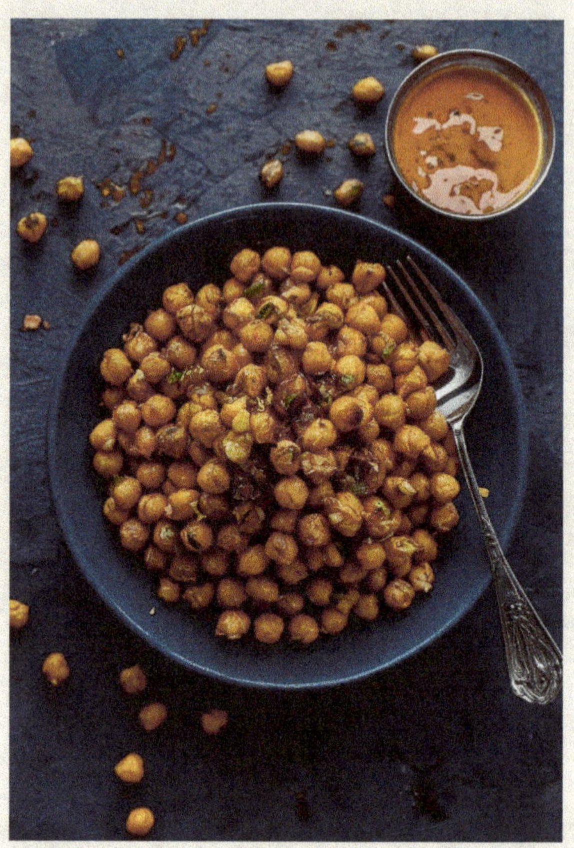

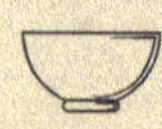 **Preparation Time : 10 min**

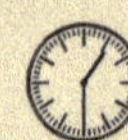 **Total Time : 50 min**

 **Servings : 4**

Nutritional Info

- Calories: 120
- Protein: 6g
- Fat: 2g
- Carbohydrates: 20g
- Fiber: 6g

BAKED KALE CHIPS

Ingredients

- 1 bunch of kale
- 1 tablespoon olive oil (optional)
- 1 teaspoon sea salt

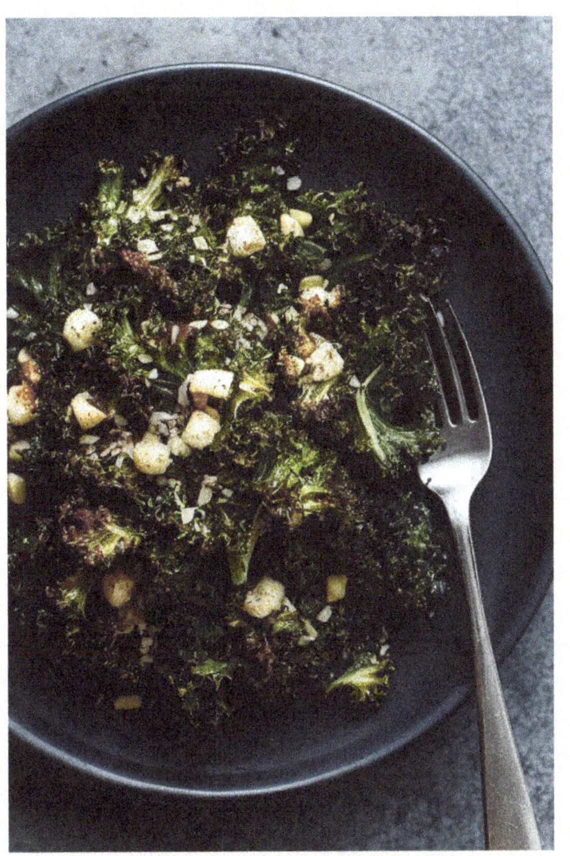

Instructions

- Preheat oven to 300°F (150°C).
- Prepare kale: Wash and dry kale. Tear into bite-sized pieces, removing stems.
- Season: Toss kale with olive oil (if using) and salt.
- Bake: Spread kale on a baking sheet in a single layer. Bake for 20 minutes, until edges are brown.
- Cool and serve: Let cool for a few minutes to crisp up. Enjoy!

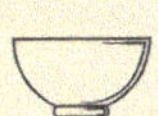 **Preparation Time : 10 min**

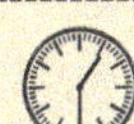 **Total Time : 30 min**

 **Servings : 4**

Nutritional Info

- Calories: 50
- Total Fat: 2g (with olive oil)
- Saturated Fat: 0g
- Cholesterol: 0mg
- Sodium: 200mg
- Total Carbohydrates: 8g

SPICED NUTS

Ingredients

- 2 cups mixed nuts (such as almonds, walnuts, and cashews)
- 1 tablespoon olive oil
- 1 tablespoon honey or maple syrup
- 1 teaspoon ground cinnamon
- 1/2 teaspoon ground nutmeg
- 1/4 teaspoon ground cloves
- 1/4 teaspoon salt

Instructions

- Preheat your oven to 350°F (175°C) and line a baking sheet with parchment paper.
- In a large bowl, combine the mixed nuts, olive oil, honey or maple syrup, cinnamon, nutmeg, cloves, and salt. Toss until the nuts are evenly coated.
- Spread the coated nuts in a single layer on the prepared baking sheet.
- Bake for 10-15 minutes, stirring occasionally, until the nuts are toasted and fragrant.
- Remove from the oven and let cool completely before serving or storing in an airtight container.

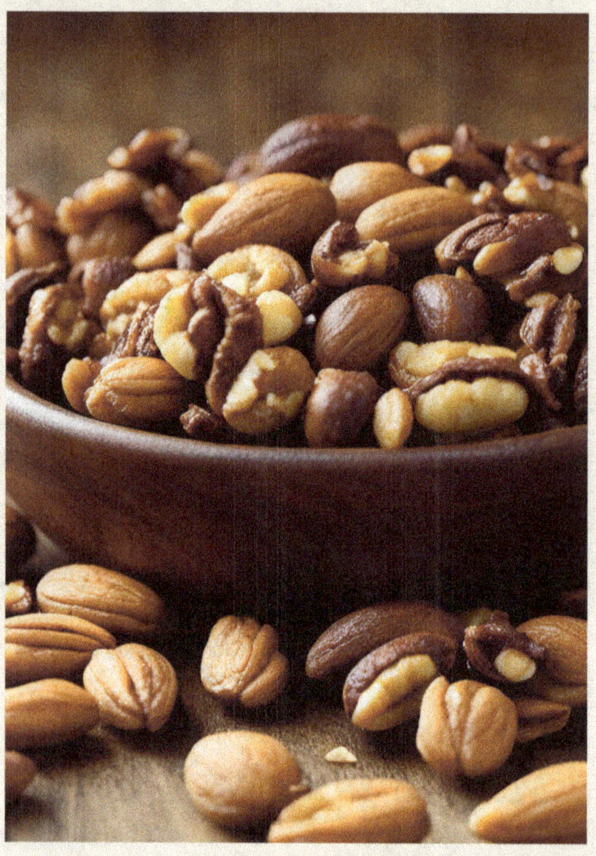

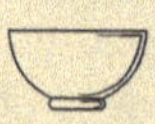 **Preparation Time : 5 min**

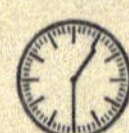 **Total Time : 20 min**

 **Servings : 1/4 cup**

Nutritional Info

- Calories: 180
- Protein: 5g
- Fat: 15g
- Carbohydrates: 8g
- Fiber: 2g

CRUNCHY CELERY AND APPLE SALAD

Ingredients

- 4 stalks of celery, thinly sliced
- 2 large apples (Granny Smith or Honeycrisp), cored and diced
- 1/4 cup walnuts, chopped (optional)
- 1/4 cup raisins (optional)
- 2 tablespoons lemon juice
- 1/2 teaspoon salt
- 1/4 teaspoon black pepper
- 1 tablespoon olive oil (optional)

Instructions

- Wash and thinly slice the celery stalks.
- Core and dice the apples into bite-sized pieces.
- In a large mixing bowl, combine the sliced celery and diced apples.
- If using, add the chopped walnuts and raisins to the bowl.
- Drizzle the lemon juice over the salad mixture to prevent the apples from browning.
- Season with salt and black pepper.
- Add the olive oil, if desired, for a richer flavor.
- Toss all ingredients together until well combined.
- Garnish with chopped parsley if desired.
- Serve the salad immediately to maintain its crunchiness.

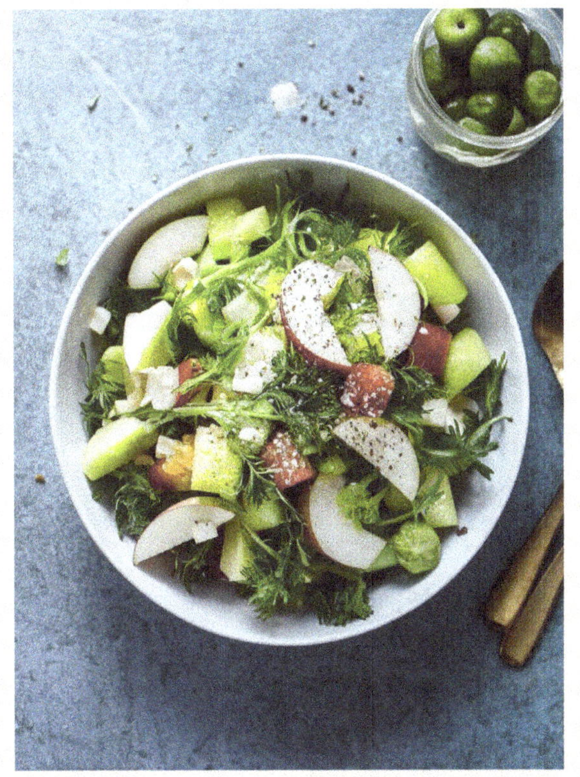

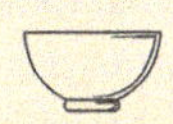 **Preparation Time : 15 min**

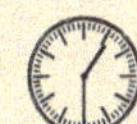 **Total Time : 15 min**

 **Servings : 4**

Nutritional Info

- Calories: 80
- Protein: 1g
- Carbohydrates: 18g
- Fat: 1g
- Fiber: 4g

MIXED BERRY SALAD

Ingredients

- 2 cups mixed berries (such as strawberries, blueberries, raspberries)
- 2 tablespoons honey
- 1 tablespoon balsamic vinegar
- 1/4 cup fresh mint leaves, chopped
- 1/4 cup crumbled feta cheese (optional)
- Salt and pepper to taste

Instructions

- Wash the berries and pat them dry. Slice the strawberries if they are large.
- In a small bowl, whisk together the honey and balsamic vinegar.
- In a large bowl, combine the mixed berries and chopped mint leaves.
- Drizzle the honey-balsamic dressing over the berries and gently toss to coat.
- Season with salt and pepper to taste.
- Sprinkle the crumbled feta cheese on top, if using.
- Serve immediately.

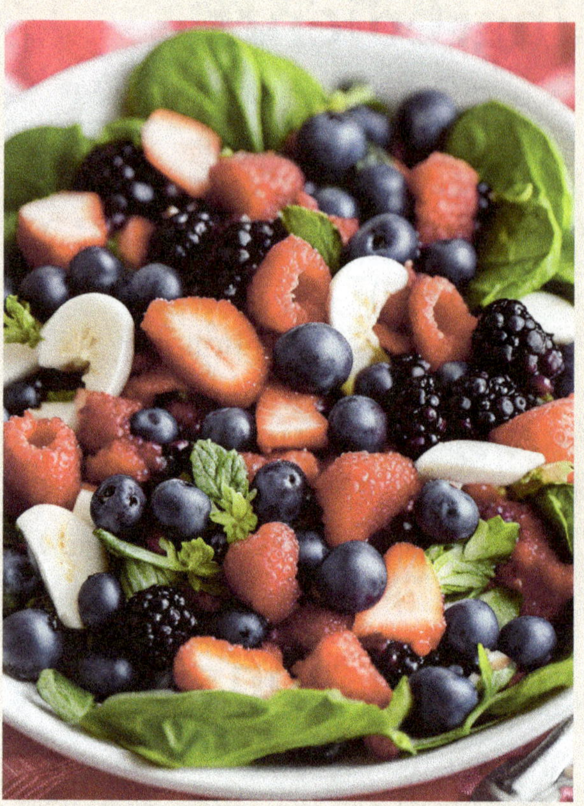

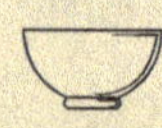 **Preparation Time : 10 min**

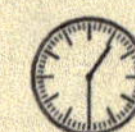 **Total Time : 10 min**

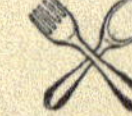 **Servings : 4**

Nutritional Info

- Calories: 90
- Total Fat: 1g
- Cholesterol: 0mg
- Sodium: 20mg
- Total Carbohydrates: 22g

ALMOND BUTTER AND APPLE SLICES

Ingredients

- 2 medium-sized apples
- 1/4 cup almond butter
- Optional: drizzle of honey or sprinkle of cinnamon

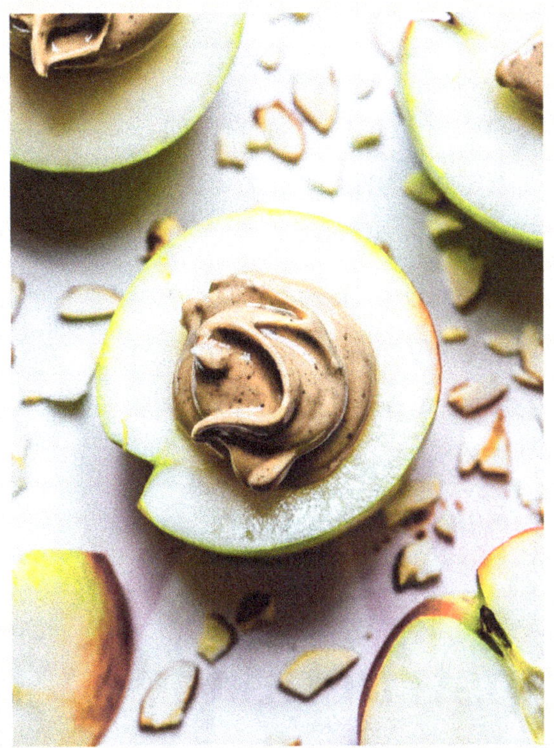

Instructions

- Wash and core the apples. Slice them into thin rounds or wedges.
- Spread almond butter on one side of each apple slice.
- Optional: Drizzle honey or sprinkle cinnamon over the almond butter.
- Serve immediately and enjoy!

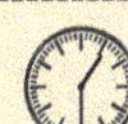 **Preparation Time : 5 min**

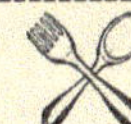 **Total Time : 5 min**

Servings : 4

Nutritional Info

- Calories: Approximately 180 kcal
- Total Fat: 11g
- Saturated Fat: 1g
- Trans Fat: 0g
- Cholesterol: 0mg
- Sodium: 5mg

MARINATED MUSHROOM SKEWERS

Ingredients

- 1 lb (450g) button mushrooms, cleaned and stems trimmed
- 2 tbsp olive oil
- 3 tbsp balsamic vinegar
- 2 cloves garlic, minced
- 1 tsp dried thyme
- 1 tsp dried rosemary
- Salt and pepper to taste

Instructions

- Mix olive oil, balsamic vinegar, garlic, thyme, rosemary, salt, and pepper in a bowl.
- Add mushrooms and toss to coat. Let sit for 10 minutes.
- If using wooden skewers, soak them in water for 10 minutes.
- Thread mushrooms onto skewers.
- Preheat grill to medium-high.
- Grill skewers for 5-7 minutes per side, until mushrooms are tender.
- Remove from grill and enjoy warm.

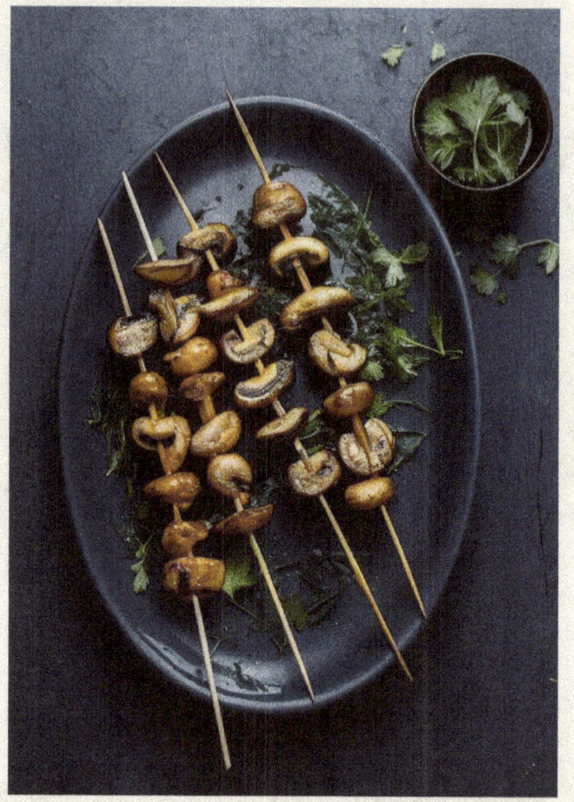

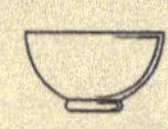 **Preparation Time : 10 min**

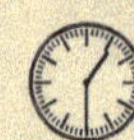 **Total Time : 20 min**

 **Servings : 4**

Nutritional Info

- Calories: 80
- Protein: 2g
- Carbohydrates: 6g
- Fat: 5g
- Fiber: 2g
- Sugar: 3g

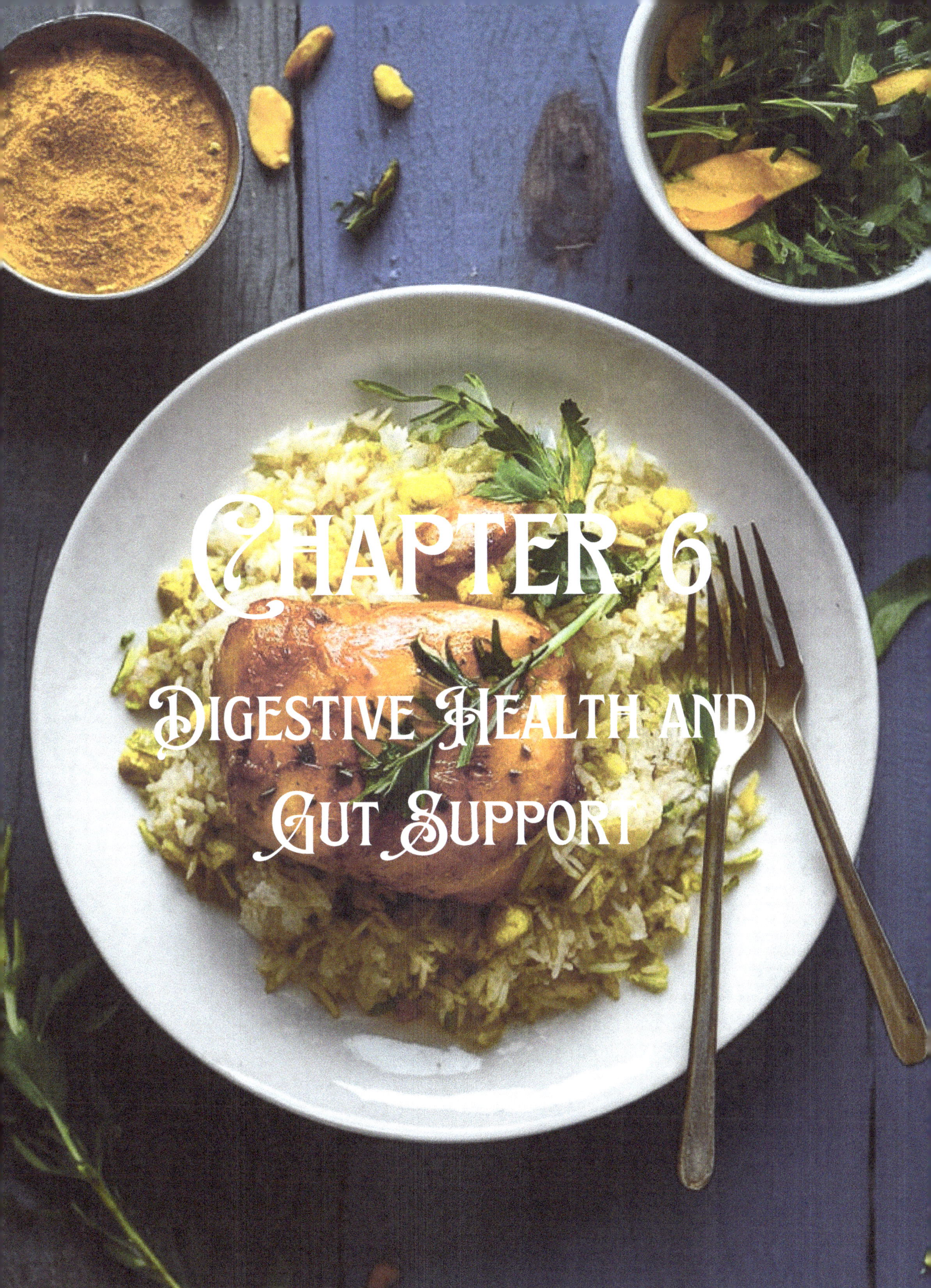

Chapter 6
Digestive Health and Gut Support

BEEF AND BROCCOLI STIR-FRY

Ingredients

- 1 lb (450g) lean beef steak, thinly sliced
- 2 cups broccoli florets
- 1 red bell pepper, thinly sliced
- 1 onion, thinly sliced
- 3 cloves garlic, minced
- 2 tbsp low-sodium soy sauce
- 1 tbsp oyster sauce
- 1 tbsp sesame oil
- 1 tbsp cornstarch
- 1 tsp fresh ginger, grated
- 2 tbsp vegetable oil
- Salt and pepper, to taste

Instructions

- In a bowl, mix soy sauce, oyster sauce, sesame oil, cornstarch, and grated ginger.
- Add beef to the marinade and let it sit for 10 minutes.
- Heat vegetable oil in a skillet or wok over medium-high heat.
- Add minced garlic and cook until fragrant, about 30 seconds.
- Add marinated beef and cook until browned, about 3 minutes. Remove beef.
- In the same skillet, add more oil if needed, then add broccoli, bell pepper, and onion. Cook for 3-4 minutes until tender-crisp.
- Return beef to the skillet, stir together, and cook for 2 minutes to heat through.
- Season with salt and pepper.
- Garnish with sesame seeds and green onions if desired.
- Serve hot over rice or noodles.

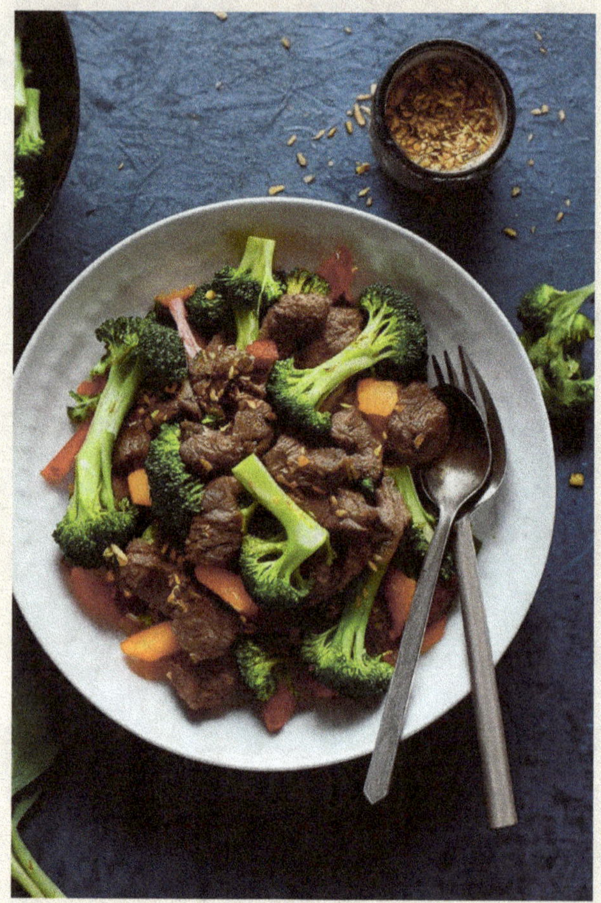

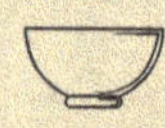
Preparation Time : 15 min

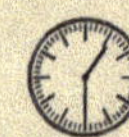
Total Time : 30 min

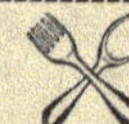
Servings : 4

Nutritional Info

- Calories: 250
- Protein: 25g
- Carbohydrates: 12g
- Fat: 11g
- Fiber: 4g

TURKEY MEATBALLS WITH ZOODLES

Ingredients

- 1 lb ground turkey
- 1/4 cup grated Parmesan cheese
- 1 large egg
- 2 cloves garlic, minced
- 1/4 cup chopped parsley
- 1 tsp dried oregano
- 1/2 tsp salt
- 1/4 tsp black pepper
- 4 medium zucchinis, spiralized
- 2 tbsp olive oil
- 1 clove garlic, minced
- Salt and pepper to taste

Instructions

- Mix turkey, Parmesan, egg, minced garlic, parsley, oregano, salt, and pepper in a bowl.
- Shape into 1-inch meatballs.
- Heat a large skillet over medium-high heat with a bit of olive oil.
- Cook meatballs until browned and cooked through, about 10-12 minutes.
- Remove meatballs from the skillet.
- In the same skillet, heat 2 tbsp olive oil over medium heat.
- Add minced garlic and cook for 1 minute.
- Add spiralized zucchini and cook for 3-5 minutes until tender.
- Season with salt and pepper.
- Return meatballs to the skillet and add marinara sauce.
- Heat until warm.
- Serve meatballs and sauce over zoodles.

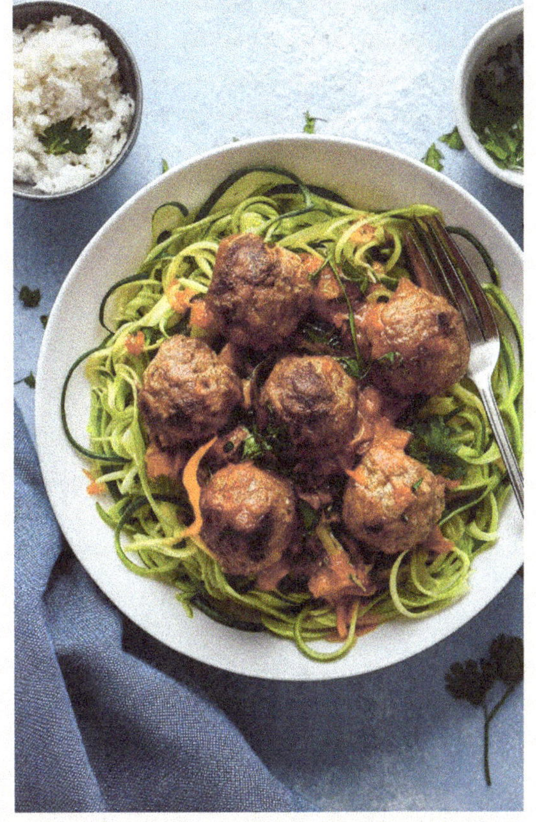

Preparation Time : 20 min

Total Time : 45 min

Servings : 4

Nutritional Info

- Calories: 250
- Protein: 30g
- Carbohydrates: 10g
- Fat: 10g
- Fiber: 3g

VEGGIE STIR-FRY WITH TOFU

Ingredients

- 1 block (14 oz) firm tofu, cubed
- 2 tablespoons soy sauce (low sodium)
- 1 tablespoon olive oil
- 2 bell peppers, sliced
- 1 cup broccoli florets
- 1 cup snap peas
- 2 cloves garlic, minced
- 1 tablespoon fresh ginger, grated
- 2 tablespoons vegetable broth (low sodium)
- Salt and pepper to taste

Instructions

- Drain, pat dry, and cube the tofu. Toss with 1 tablespoon soy sauce.
- Heat olive oil in a large pan over medium-high heat. Cook tofu until golden brown, about 5-7 minutes. Remove from pan.
- In the same pan, add garlic and ginger, sauté for 30 seconds.
- Add bell peppers, broccoli, and snap peas. Stir-fry for 4-5 minutes until tender-crisp.
- Return tofu to pan. Add 1 tablespoon soy sauce and vegetable broth. Stir and cook for 2-3 minutes.
- Season with salt and pepper. Serve warm.

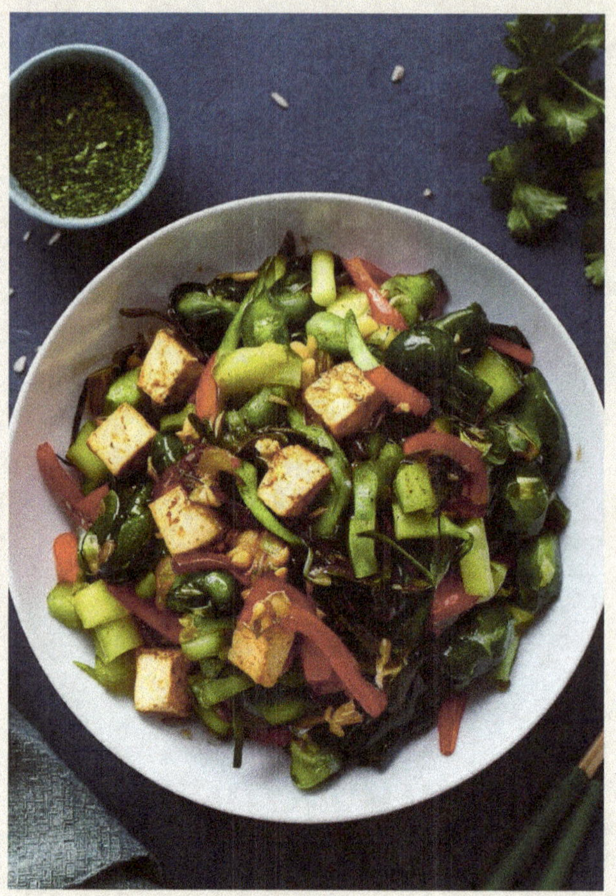

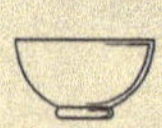 **Preparation Time : 10 min**

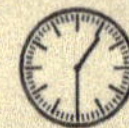 **Total Time : 20 min**

 **Servings : 4**

Nutritional Info

- Calories: 180
- Protein: 12g
- Carbohydrates: 16g
- Fat: 8g
- Fiber: 5g

HERB-CRUSTED CHICKEN BREAST

Ingredients

- 4 boneless, skinless chicken breasts
- 2 tablespoons olive oil
- 1/4 cup fresh parsley, chopped
- 1/4 cup fresh basil, chopped
- 1/4 cup fresh thyme, chopped
- 2 cloves garlic, minced
- 1 teaspoon salt
- 1/2 teaspoon black pepper
- 1 teaspoon lemon zest

Instructions

- Preheat Oven: Preheat your oven to 400°F (200°C).
- Prepare Herb Mixture: In a small bowl, combine the chopped parsley, basil, thyme, minced garlic, salt, black pepper, and lemon zest.
- Prepare Chicken: Pat the chicken breasts dry with paper towels. Rub each breast with olive oil, ensuring they are evenly coated.
- Coat with Herbs: Press the herb mixture onto both sides of each chicken breast, making sure they are well coated.
- Bake Chicken: Place the chicken breasts on a baking sheet lined with parchment paper or in a lightly greased baking dish.
- Cook: Bake in the preheated oven for 25 minutes, or until the internal temperature of the chicken reaches 165°F (74°C) and the exterior is golden brown.
- Rest and Serve: Let the chicken rest for 5 minutes before serving to allow the juices to redistribute.

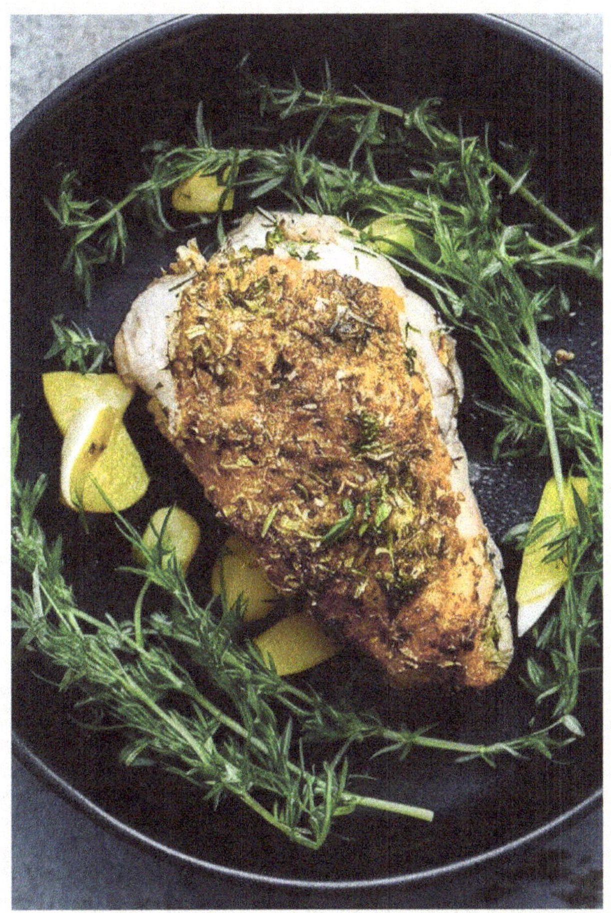

Preparation Time : 15 min

Total Time : 40 min

Servings : 4

Nutritional Info

- Calories: 220
- Protein: 28g
- Carbohydrates: 2g
- Fat: 11g

SPAGHETTI SQUASH WITH MARINARA SAUCE

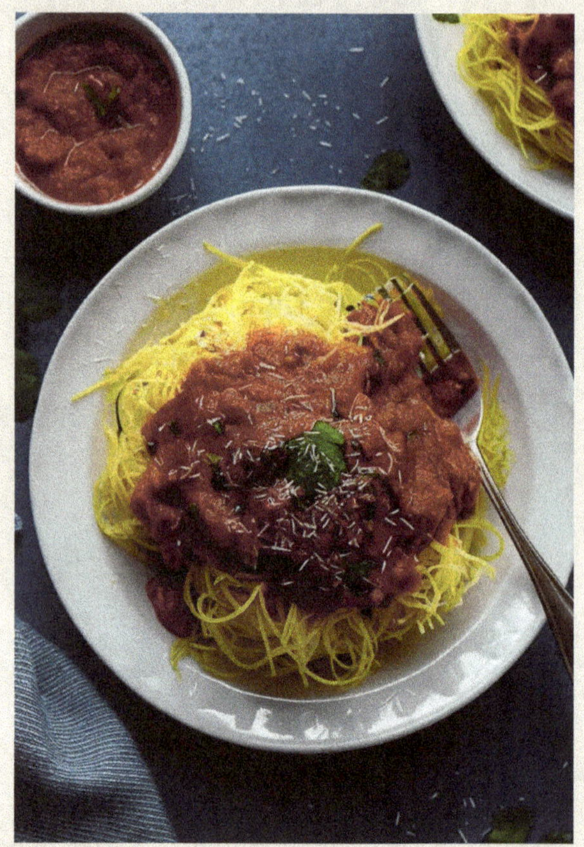

Ingredients

- 1 medium spaghetti squash
- 2 cups marinara sauce
- 2 tablespoons olive oil
- Salt and pepper to taste

Instructions

- Preheat oven to 400°F (200°C).
- Cut spaghetti squash in half lengthwise and remove seeds.
- Drizzle olive oil over cut sides of squash and season with salt and pepper.
- Place squash halves cut-side down on a baking sheet.
- Roast squash in oven for 35-40 minutes, until tender.
- While squash is roasting, heat marinara sauce in a saucepan on medium heat.
- Once squash is done, remove from oven and let cool slightly.
- Use a fork to scrape flesh into spaghetti-like strands onto a plate.
- Pour heated marinara sauce over spaghetti squash.
- Serve hot and enjoy!

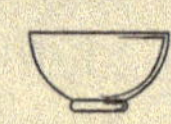 **Preparation Time : 10 min**

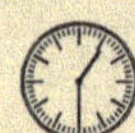 **Total Time : 50 min**

 **Servings : 4**

Nutritional Info

- Calories: 150
- Total Fat: 6g
- Total Carbohydrates: 24g
- Protein: 3g

BALSAMIC GLAZED CHICKEN BREAST

Ingredients

- 4 boneless, skinless chicken breasts
- 1/2 cup balsamic vinegar
- 2 tablespoons honey
- 2 cloves garlic, minced
- 1 teaspoon dried thyme
- Salt and pepper
- 1 tablespoon olive oil

Instructions

- Mix balsamic vinegar, honey, minced garlic, and dried thyme in a bowl.
- Pour over chicken breasts and let sit for 10 minutes.
- Heat olive oil in a skillet over medium-high heat.
- Remove chicken from marinade (save marinade) and season with salt and pepper.
- Cook chicken for 5 minutes on each side until browned.
- Pour the reserved marinade into the skillet.
- Cook for another 10 minutes, turning chicken to coat with glaze, until chicken is cooked through (165°F internal temperature).
- Let chicken rest for 5 minutes.
- Drizzle with remaining glaze from the skillet.

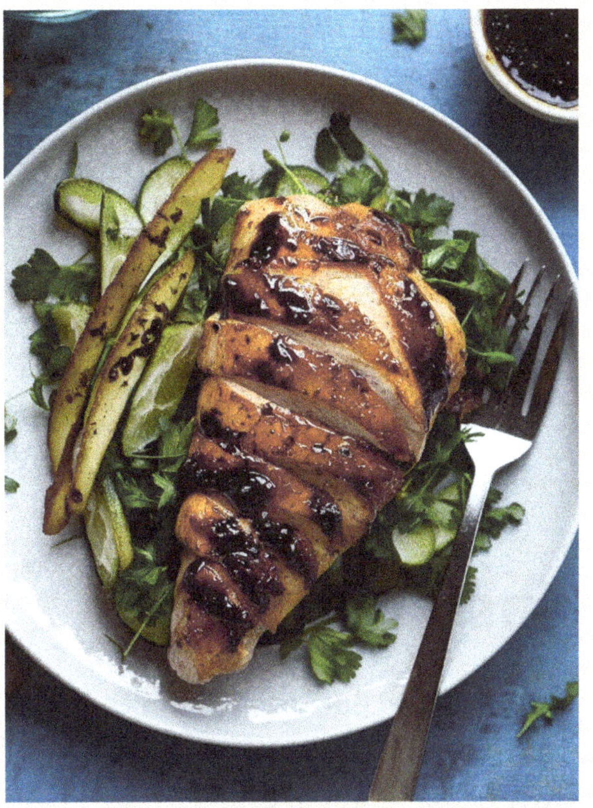

Preparation Time : 10 min

Total Time : 30 min

Servings : 4

Nutritional Info

- Calories: 200
- Protein: 30g
- Fat: 4g
- Carbohydrates: 8g

GRILLED VEGETABLE KEBABS

Ingredients

- 1 red bell pepper, cut into chunks
- 1 yellow bell pepper, cut into chunks
- 1 zucchini, sliced into rounds
- 1 red onion, cut into chunks
- 8 cherry tomatoes
- 8 button mushrooms
- 2 tablespoons olive oil
- 1 teaspoon dried oregano
- 1 teaspoon dried basil
- Salt and pepper to taste

Instructions

- Wash and cut the vegetables as indicated.
- If using wooden skewers, soak them in water for at least 10 minutes to prevent burning.
- In a large bowl, combine the olive oil, dried oregano, dried basil, salt, and pepper.
- Add the cut vegetables to the bowl and toss to coat them evenly with the marinade.
- Thread the marinated vegetables onto the skewers, alternating between different types of vegetables for a colorful presentation.
- Preheat your grill to medium-high heat.
- Place the kebabs on the preheated grill.
- Grill for about 10-15 minutes, turning occasionally, until the vegetables are tender and slightly charred.
- Remove the kebabs from the grill and serve immediately.

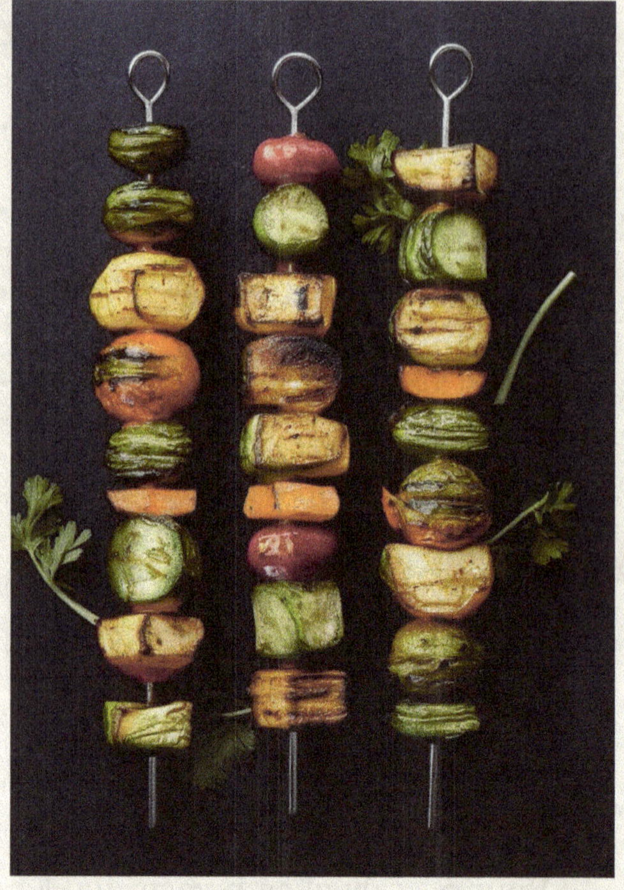

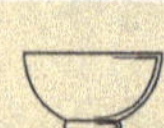
Preparation Time : 20 min

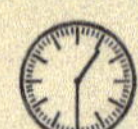
Total Time : 35min

Servings : 4

Nutritional Info

- Calories: 90
- Protein: 3g
- Carbohydrates: 15g
- Fat: 3g
- Fiber: 5g

BAKED COD WITH LEMON AND DILL

Ingredients

- 4 cod fillets (about 6 ounces each)
- 2 tablespoons olive oil
- 2 cloves garlic, minced
- 1 tablespoon fresh dill, chopped
- 1 lemon, thinly sliced
- Salt and pepper to taste

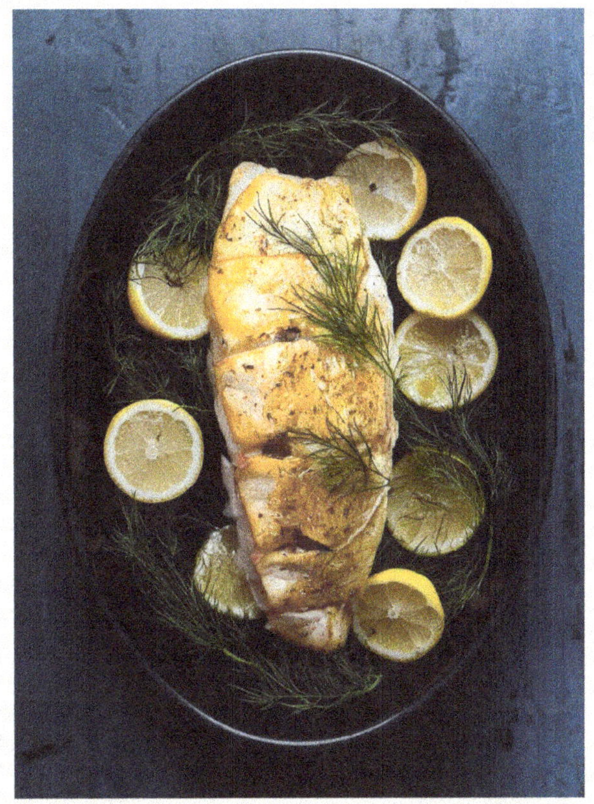

Instructions

- Preheat your oven to 375°F (190°C).
- Place the cod fillets on a baking dish lined with parchment paper or lightly greased.
- In a small bowl, mix together the olive oil, minced garlic, and chopped dill.
- Drizzle the olive oil mixture over the cod fillets, making sure they are evenly coated.
- Season the cod fillets with salt and pepper to taste.
- Place lemon slices on top of each cod fillet.
- Bake in the preheated oven for about 15-20 minutes, or until the cod is cooked through and flakes easily with a fork.
- Remove from the oven cod serve hot, garnished with additional fresh dill if desired.

Preparation Time : 10 min

Total Time : 30 min

Servings : 4

Nutritional Info

- Calories: 150 kcal
- Protein: 25g
- Carbohydrates: 2g
- Fat: 4g
- Fiber: 0.5g
- Sugar: 0g

BAKED LEMON HERB SALMON

Ingredients

- 4 salmon fillets (about 6 oz each)
- 2 tablespoons olive oil
- 2 lemons (one for juice, one for slices)
- 3 cloves garlic, minced
- 2 tablespoons fresh parsley, chopped
- 1 tablespoon fresh dill, chopped
- 1 teaspoon salt
- 1/2 teaspoon black pepper

Instructions

- Preheat your oven to 400°F (200°C).
- Place the salmon fillets on a baking sheet lined with parchment paper.
- In a small bowl, mix the olive oil, juice of one lemon, minced garlic, chopped parsley, chopped dill, salt, and black pepper.
- Brush the marinade generously over each salmon fillet. Let it sit for about 10 minutes to allow the flavors to infuse.
- Slice the second lemon into thin rounds and place a couple of slices on top of each salmon fillet.
- Bake in the preheated oven for 20 minutes, or until the salmon is cooked through and flakes easily with a fork.
- Remove from the oven and transfer to plates. Serve immediately, optionally garnished with extra fresh herbs and lemon wedges.

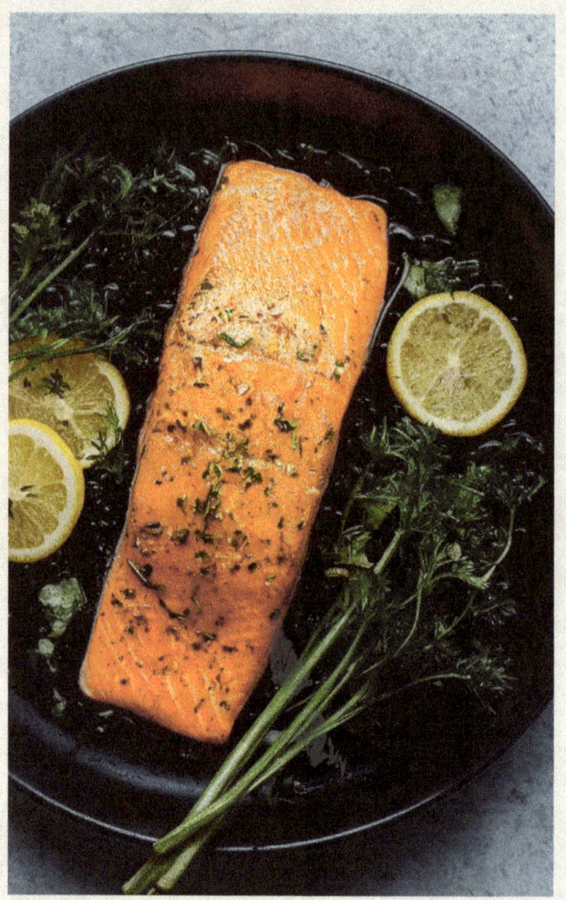

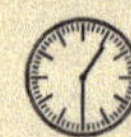 **Preparation Time : 10 min**

 **Total Time : 30 min**

Servings : 4

Nutritional Info

- Calories: 230
- Protein: 25g
- Fat: 14g
- Carbohydrates: 2g
- Fiber: 1g

GRILLED SHRIMP SKEWERS

Ingredients

- 1 lb large shrimp, peeled and deveined
- 2 cloves garlic, minced
- 2 tbsp olive oil
- 1 tbsp lemon juice
- 1 tsp smoked paprika
- Salt and pepper to taste
- Fresh parsley, chopped (for garnish)

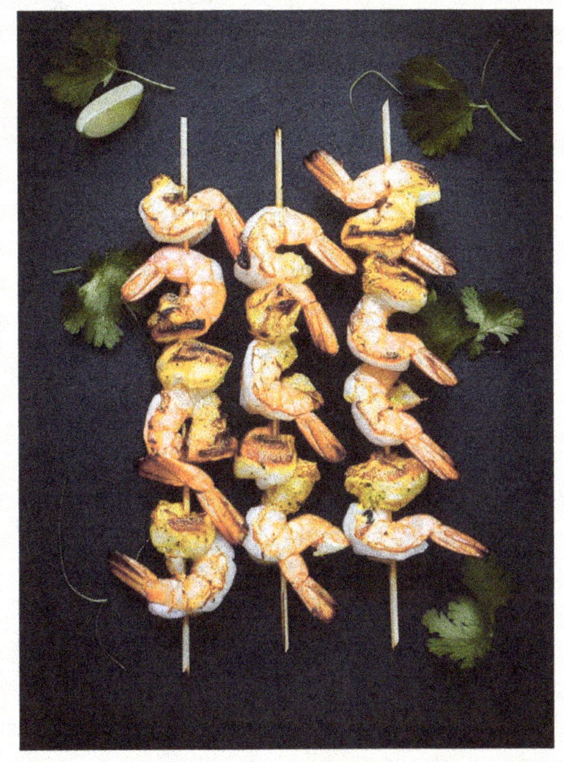

Instructions

- Marinate the Shrimp: In a large bowl, combine minced garlic, olive oil, lemon juice, smoked paprika, salt, and pepper. Add the shrimp and toss to coat. Let it marinate for 10 minutes.
- Prepare the Skewers: If using wooden skewers, soak them in water for 10 minutes to prevent burning. Thread the shrimp onto the skewers, leaving a little space between each shrimp.
- Preheat the Grill: Preheat the grill to medium-high heat.
- Grill the Shrimp: Place the shrimp skewers on the grill. Cook for 2-3 minutes per side, until the shrimp are opaque and cooked through.
- Serve: Remove the skewers from the grill and transfer to a serving platter. Garnish with chopped fresh parsley and lemon wedges. Serve immediately.

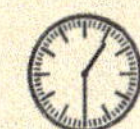 **Preparation Time : 15 min**

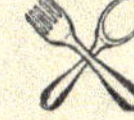 **Total Time : 25 min**

Servings : 4

Nutritional Info

- Calories: 150
- Protein: 23g
- Carbohydrates: 2g
- Fat: 6g
- Fiber: 0g

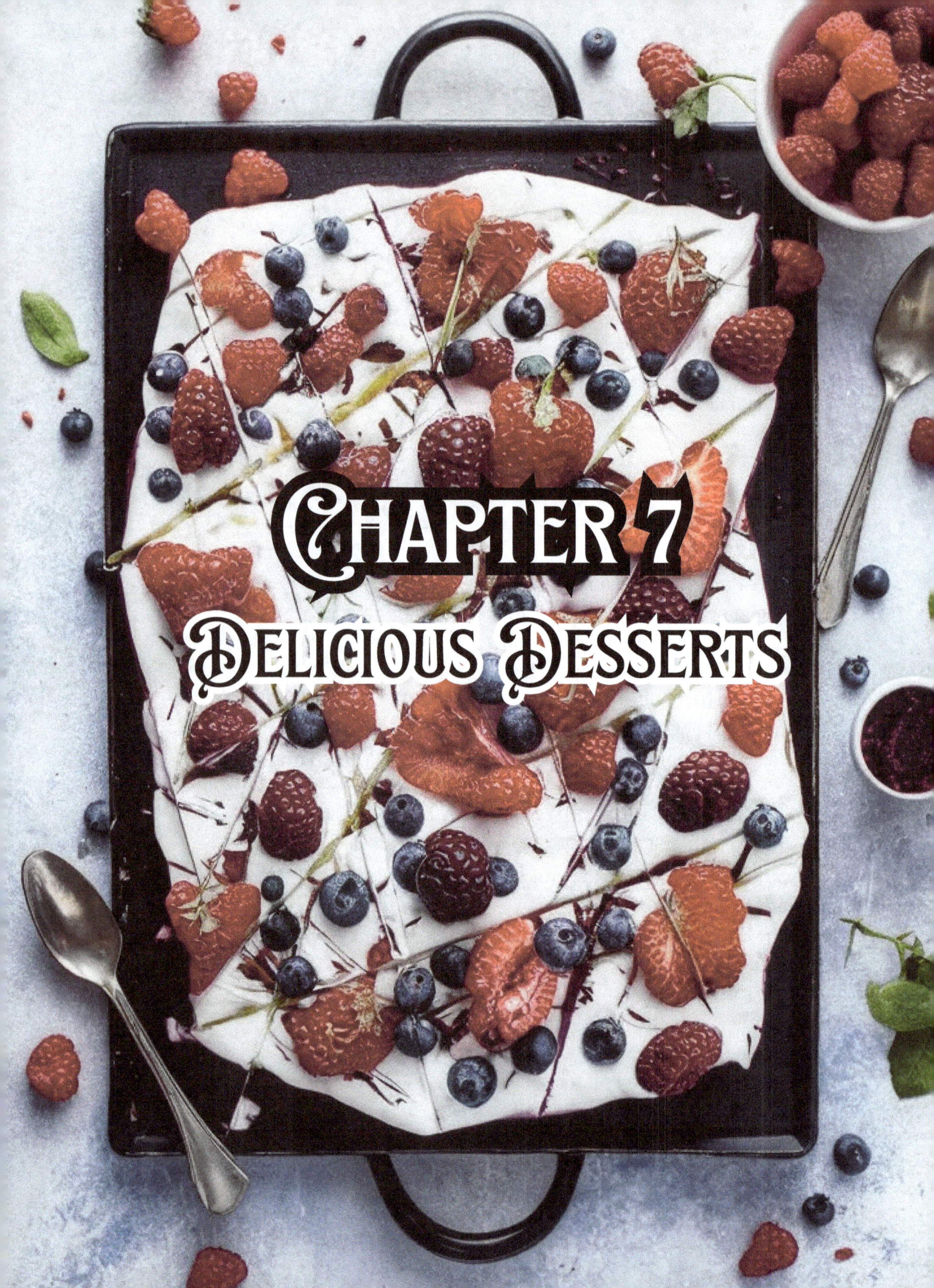

Chapter 7
Delicious Desserts

MIXED BERRY SORBET

Ingredients

- 3 cups mixed berries (such as strawberries, blueberries, raspberries)
- 1/4 cup honey or maple syrup (optional)
- 2 tablespoons lemon juice

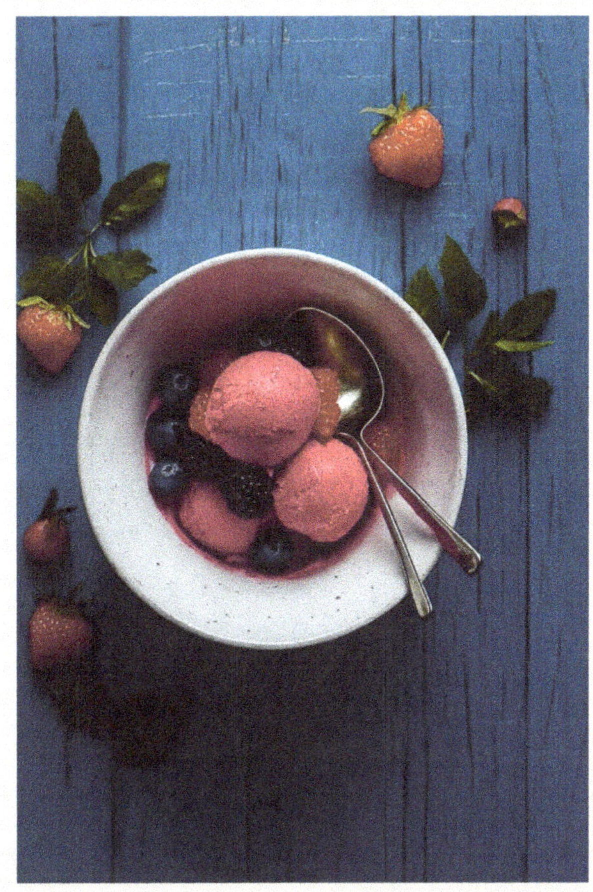

Instructions

- Blend: Put the mixed berries, honey or maple syrup (if using), and lemon juice in a blender or food processor.
- Blend Again: Blend until smooth.
- Freeze: Pour the mixture into a shallow dish or pan. Cover and freeze for 3-4 hours, or until partially frozen.
- Scrape and Blend: Once partially frozen, scrape the mixture with a fork to break it up into icy flakes. Blend again until smooth.
- Freeze Again: Return the mixture to the dish or pan. Cover and freeze for another 2-3 hours, or until firm.
- Serve: Scoop the sorbet into bowls or glasses.
- Enjoy: Garnish with fresh mint leaves if desired, then serve and enjoy!

Preparation Time : 10 min

Total Time : 0 min

Servings : 4

Nutritional Info

- Calories: Approximately 80 kcal
- Carbohydrates: Approximately 20 g
- Fiber: Approximately 3 g
- Sugars: Approximately 15 g
- Fat: Approximately 0 g

APPLE CINNAMON COMPOTE

Ingredients

- 4 medium apples, peeled, cored, and chopped
- 1 tablespoon lemon juice
- 1/4 cup water
- 2 tablespoons honey or maple syrup (optional)
- 1 teaspoon ground cinnamon
- 1/2 teaspoon vanilla extract (optional)

Instructions

- In a medium saucepan, combine the chopped apples, lemon juice, and water.
- Bring the mixture to a simmer over medium heat.
- Stir in the honey or maple syrup (if using), ground cinnamon, and vanilla extract (if using).
- Reduce the heat to low and let the mixture cook uncovered for about 15-20 minutes, or until the apples are soft and the liquid has thickened slightly, stirring occasionally.
- Once the apples are cooked to your desired consistency, remove the saucepan from the heat.
- Allow the compote to cool slightly before serving. You can serve it warm or chilled, depending on your preference.
- Enjoy the apple cinnamon compote on its own, or use it as a topping for yogurt, oatmeal, pancakes, or ice cream.

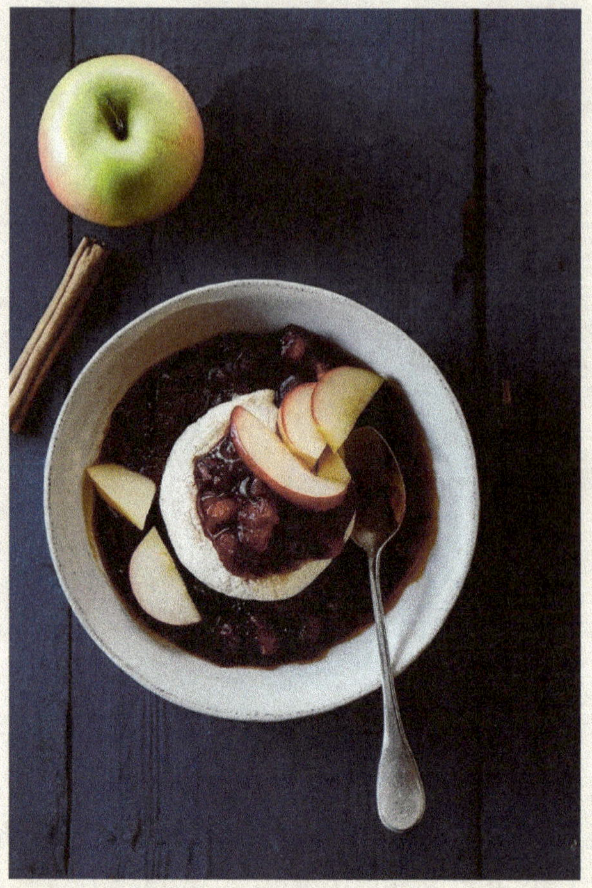

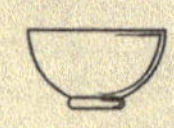
Preparation Time : 10 min

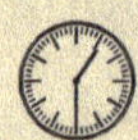
Total Time : 30 min

Servings : 4

Nutritional Info

- Calories: 80 kcal
- Carbohydrates: 20 g
- Fiber: 4 g
- Sugars: 15 g
- Fat: 0 g
- Protein: 0 g

PEACH AND RASPBERRY CRUMBLE

Ingredients

- 1 ripe peach, sliced
- 1/2 cup fresh raspberries
- 1 tablespoon lemon juice
- 2 tablespoons granulated sugar (or sweetener of choice)
- 1/4 cup rolled oats
- 2 tablespoons all-purpose flour
- 1 tablespoon brown sugar
- 1/4 teaspoon ground cinnamon
- 2 tablespoons unsalted butter, chilled and cubed

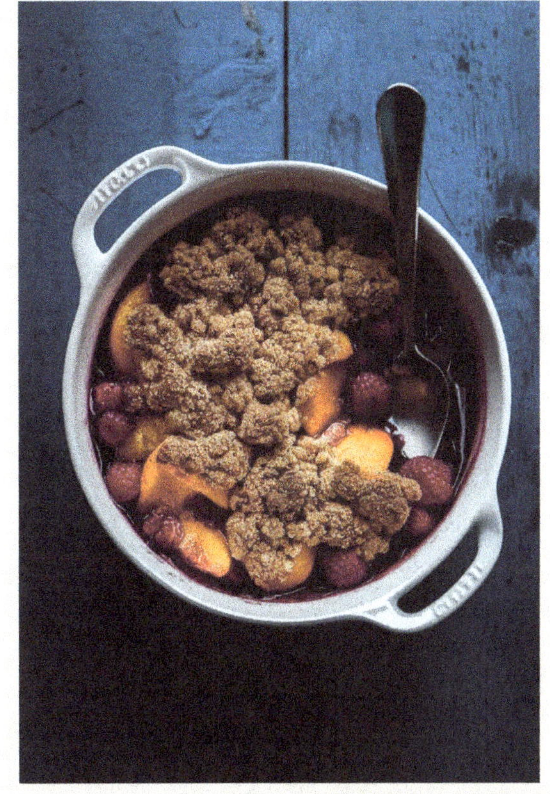

Instructions

- Preheat your oven to 375°F (190°C). Lightly grease a small baking dish or individual ramekins.
- In a bowl, toss together the sliced peach, raspberries, lemon juice, and granulated sugar until well combined. Transfer the fruit mixture to the prepared baking dish or ramekins, spreading it out evenly.
- In another bowl, mix together the rolled oats, all-purpose flour, brown sugar, and ground cinnamon.
- Using your fingers, incorporate the chilled cubed butter into the oat mixture until it resembles coarse crumbs.
- Sprinkle the oat mixture evenly over the fruit in the baking dish or ramekins.
- Place the baking dish or ramekins in the preheated oven and bake for about 25-30 minutes, or until the fruit is bubbly and the crumble topping is golden brown.
- Remove from the oven and let it cool for a few minutes before serving.
- Serve warm as is or with a scoop of vanilla frozen yogurt or a dollop of whipped cream, if desired.

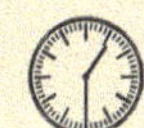 **Preparation Time : 15 min**

 **Total Time : 45 min**

Servings : 1

Nutritional Info

- Calories: 250 kcal
- Carbohydrates: 40g
- Protein: 3g
- Fat: 10g
- Fiber: 5g

BAKED APPLES WITH CINNAMON

Ingredients

- 4 medium-sized apples
- 1 teaspoon ground cinnamon

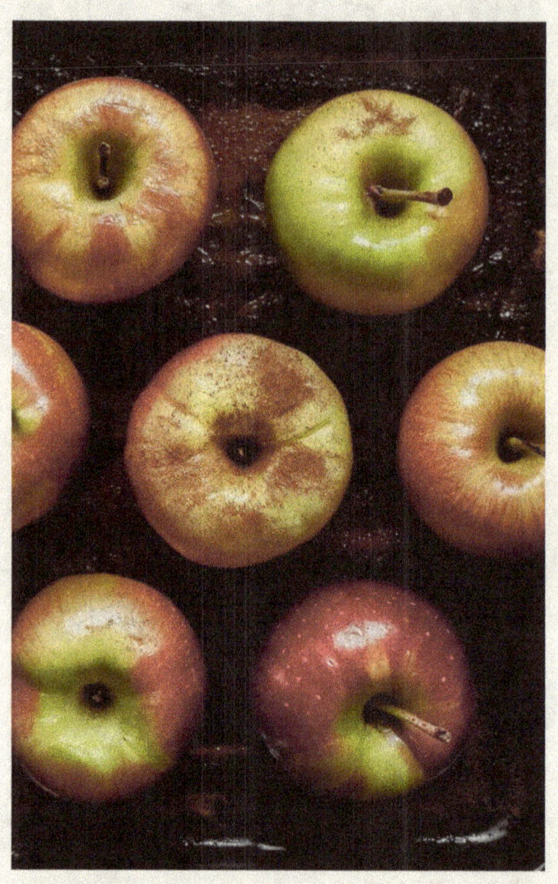

Instructions

- Preheat your oven to 375°F (190°C).
- Wash the apples and remove the cores, leaving the bottoms intact to hold the filling.
- Place the cored apples in a baking dish.
- Sprinkle ground cinnamon evenly over each apple.
- Bake for 25 minutes, or until the apples are tender.
- Serve warm as is or with a dollop of Greek yogurt or a scoop of vanilla ice cream, if desired.

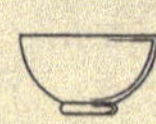 **Preparation Time : 5 min**

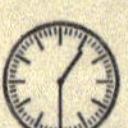 **Total Time : 30 min**

 **Servings : 4**

Nutritional Info

- Calories: 120 kcal
- Total Fat: 0.5g
- Carbohydrates: 31g
- Fiber: 5g
- Sugars: 24g
- Protein: 0.5g

BLUEBERRY AND LEMON SORBET

Ingredients

- 2 cups fresh blueberries
- 1/2 cup water
- 1/2 cup granulated sugar
- Zest and juice of 1 lemon

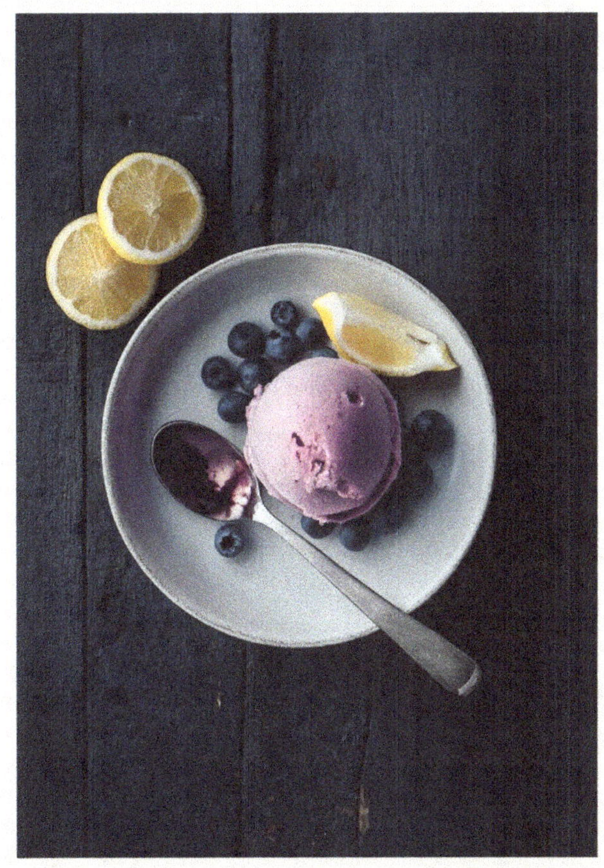

Instructions

- Combine Ingredients: In a saucepan, mix blueberries, water, and sugar. Heat on medium until sugar dissolves and blueberries soften (about 5 minutes).
- Blend: Pour mixture into a blender, add lemon zest and juice, blend until smooth.
- Strain (Optional): If desired, strain mixture through a sieve for smoother texture.
- Chill and Freeze: Cool mixture in the fridge for 2 hours. Pour into a shallow dish, freeze for 4-6 hours. Stir every hour.
- Serve: Scoop into bowls, garnish with blueberries or lemon zest. Enjoy!

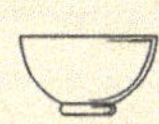 **Preparation Time : 10 min**

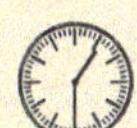 **Total Time : 15 min**

 **Servings : 4**

Nutritional Info

- Calories: 80 kcal
- Fat: 0g
- Carbohydrates: 20g
- Fiber: 3g
- Sugars: 14g
- Protein: 1g

MANGO AND PINEAPPLE SALAD

Ingredients

- 1 ripe mango, peeled and diced
- 1 cup fresh pineapple chunks
- 1/4 cup red onion, finely chopped
- 1/4 cup fresh cilantro, chopped
- Juice of 1 lime
- Salt and pepper to taste

Instructions

- In a large mixing bowl, combine the diced mango, pineapple chunks, chopped red onion, and chopped cilantro.
- Squeeze the lime juice over the fruit mixture.
- Season with salt and pepper to taste.
- Gently toss the ingredients until everything is evenly coated with lime juice and seasoning.
- Serve immediately as a refreshing side dish or as a topping for grilled chicken or fish.

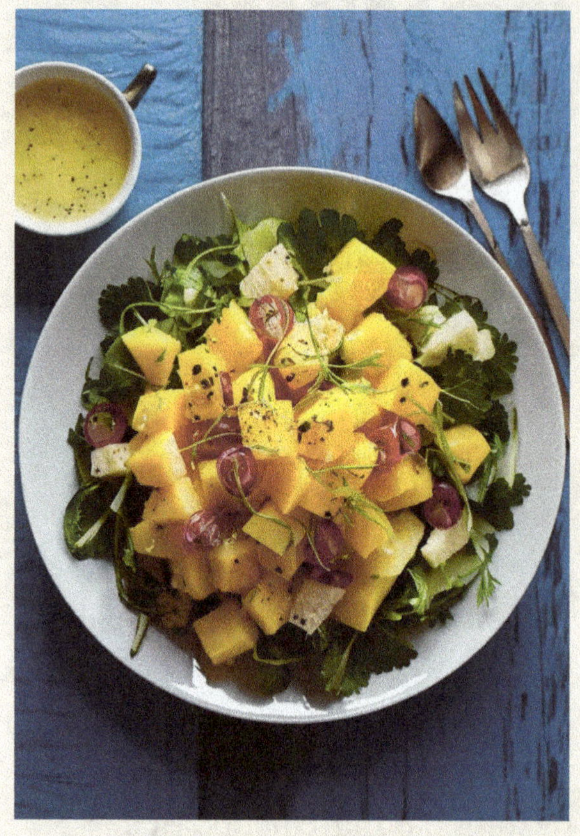

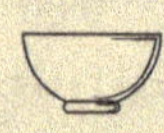 **Preparation Time : 10 min**

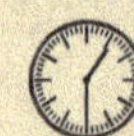 **Total Time : 0 min**

 **Servings : 4**

Nutritional Info

- Calories: 80 kcal
- Protein: 1g
- Carbohydrates: 21g
- Fat: 0g
- Fiber: 3g
- Sugar: 16g
- Sodium: 5mg

FROZEN YOGURT BARK WITH BERRIES

Ingredients

- 2 cups plain Greek yogurt
- 2 tablespoons honey or maple syrup
- 1 teaspoon vanilla extract
- 1 cup mixed berries (such as strawberries, blueberries, and raspberries)
- Optional: 2 tablespoons shredded coconut or chopped nuts for toppin

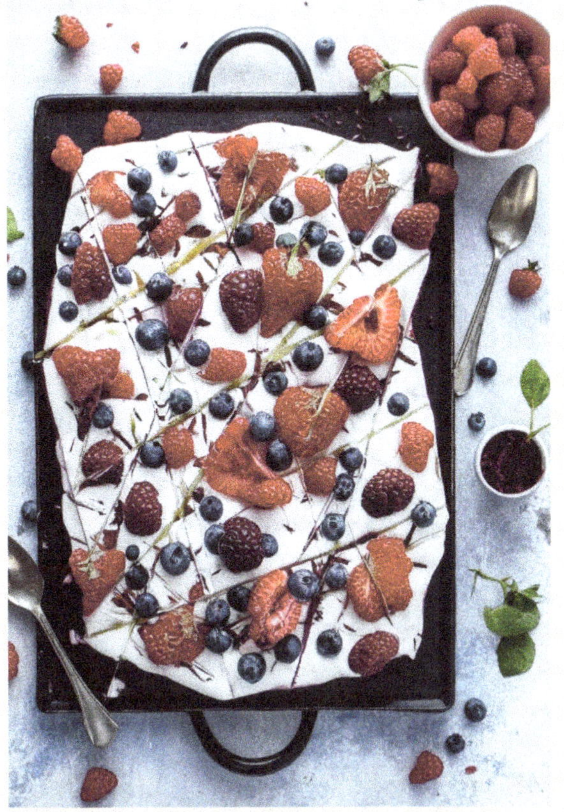

Instructions

- In a mixing bowl, combine the Greek yogurt, honey (or maple syrup), and vanilla extract. Stir until well combined.
- Line a baking sheet with parchment paper or a silicone baking mat.
- Pour the yogurt mixture onto the prepared baking sheet, spreading it evenly to about ¼ inch thickness.
- Scatter the mixed berries evenly over the yogurt mixture. Press them gently into the yogurt.
- If desired, sprinkle shredded coconut or chopped nuts over the top for added texture and flavor.
- Place the baking sheet in the freezer and let the yogurt bark freeze for at least 2 hours, or until completely firm.
- Once frozen, remove the baking sheet from the freezer and break the yogurt bark into pieces using your hands or a knife.
- Serve immediately as a refreshing snack or dessert. Store any leftovers in an airtight container in the freezer.

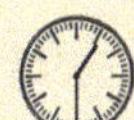 **Preparation Time : 10 min**

 **Total Time : 2hrs 10 min**

Servings : 6

Nutritional Info

- Calories: 110 kcal
- Total Fat: 2g
- Saturated Fat: 1g
- Cholesterol: 5mg
- Sodium: 25mg
- Total Carbohydrates: 14g

CHOCOLATE DIPPED STRAWBERRIES

Ingredients

- 1 pint of fresh strawberries, washed and dried
- 4 oz (about 120g) of dark chocolate chips or chopped dark chocolate (70% cocoa or higher)

Instructions

- Line a baking sheet with parchment paper.
- In a microwave-safe bowl, melt the dark chocolate chips in 30-second intervals, stirring in between, until smooth and fully melted.
- Hold each strawberry by the stem and dip it into the melted chocolate, swirling to coat it partially.
- Place the dipped strawberries onto the prepared baking sheet.
- Repeat with the remaining strawberries.
- Place the baking sheet in the refrigerator for about 15-20 minutes or until the chocolate sets.
- Once the chocolate has hardened, transfer the chocolate-dipped strawberries to a serving plate.
- Serve immediately as a delicious and healthy dessert option.

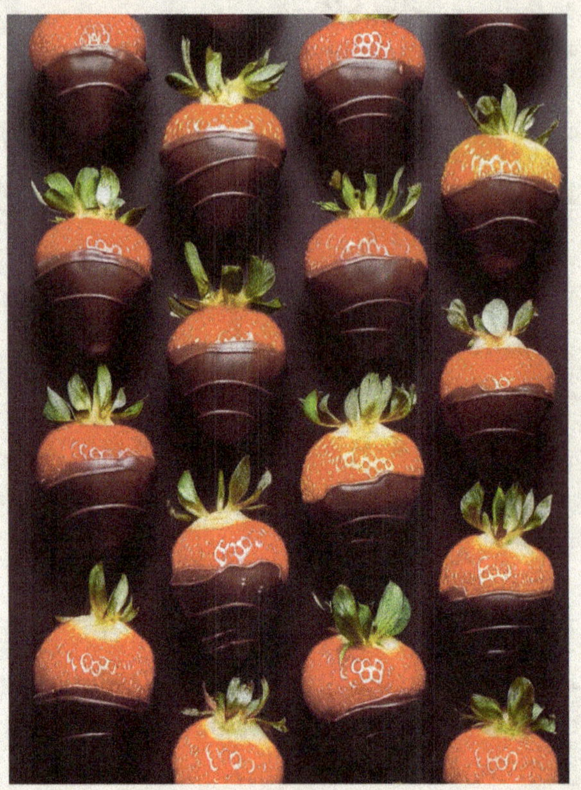

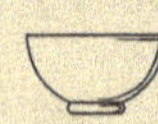 **Preparation Time : 10 min**

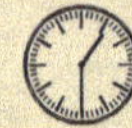 **Total Time : 15 min**

 **Servings : 4**

Nutritional Info

- Calories: 120
- Total Fat: 7g
- Saturated Fat: 4g
- Cholesterol: 0mg
- Sodium: 5mg
- Total Carbohydrates: 15g

GRILLED PINEAPPLE WITH CINNAMON

Ingredients

- 1 ripe pineapple, peeled and cored
- 1 teaspoon ground cinnamon

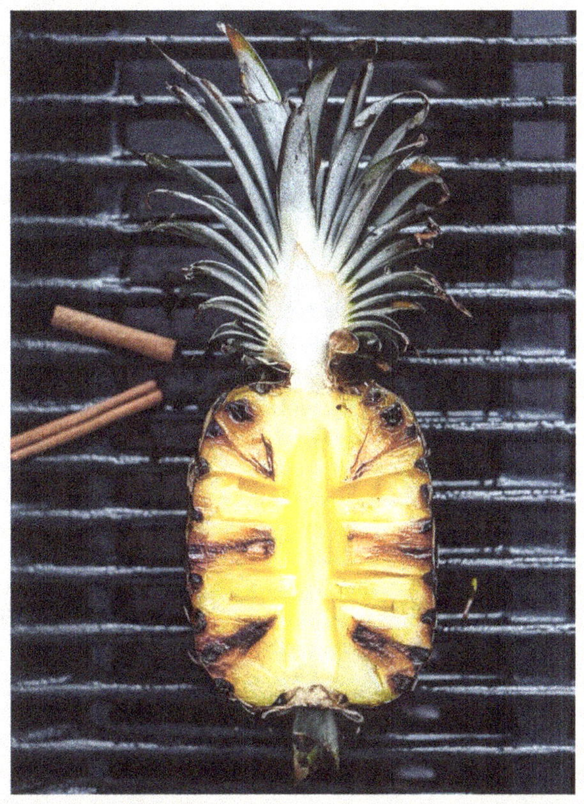

Instructions

- Preheat your grill to medium-high heat.
- Slice the pineapple into rings or wedges, about 1/2 inch thick.
- Sprinkle both sides of the pineapple slices with ground cinnamon.
- Place the pineapple slices on the preheated grill.
- Grill for 3-4 minutes on each side, or until grill marks appear and the pineapple is heated through.
- Remove from the grill and serve hot.

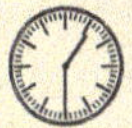 **Preparation Time : 10 min**

Total Time : 5 min

 **Servings : 2**

Nutritional Info

- Calories: 90
- Total Fat: 0g
- Saturated Fat: 0g
- Cholesterol: 0mg
- Sodium: 0mg
- Total Carbohydrates: 23g

COCONUT MACAROONS

Ingredients

- 3 cups shredded coconut
- 3/4 cup sweetened condensed milk
- 2 large egg whites
- 1 teaspoon vanilla extract
- Pinch of salt

Instructions

- Preheat your oven to 325°F (160°C). Line a baking sheet with parchment paper.
- In a large bowl, combine the shredded coconut, sweetened condensed milk, vanilla extract, and salt. Mix well until evenly combined.
- In a separate bowl, beat the egg whites until stiff peaks form.
- Gently fold the beaten egg whites into the coconut mixture until fully incorporated.
- Using a spoon or cookie scoop, drop rounded tablespoons of the mixture onto the prepared baking sheet, spacing them about 1 inch apart.
- Bake in the preheated oven for 20-25 minutes, or until the macaroons are golden brown on the edges.
- Remove from the oven and let cool on the baking sheet for a few minutes before transferring to a wire rack to cool completely.

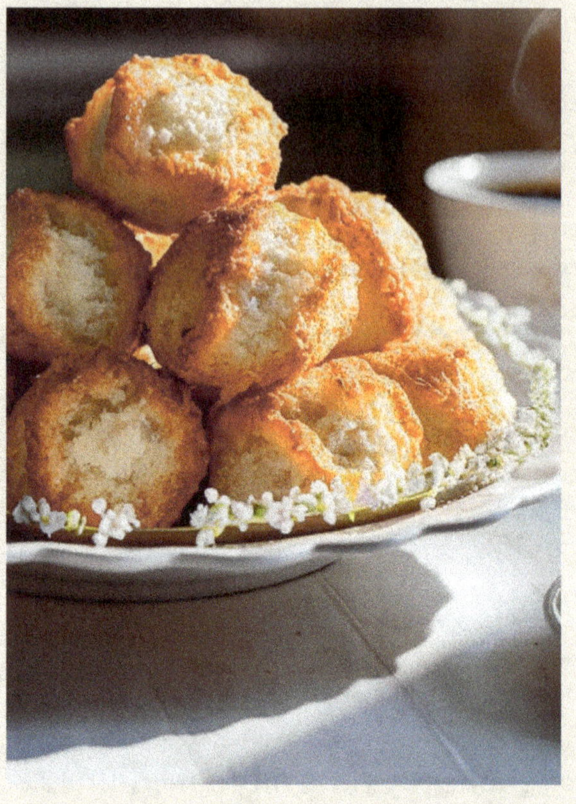

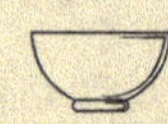 **Preparation Time : 10 min**

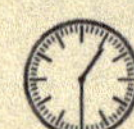 **Total Time : 35 min**

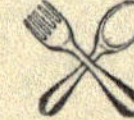 **Servings : 20 macaroons**

Nutritional Info

- Calories: 120 kcal
- Total Fat: 7g
- Saturated Fat: 6g
- Trans Fat: 0g
- Cholesterol: 3mg
- Sodium: 60mg

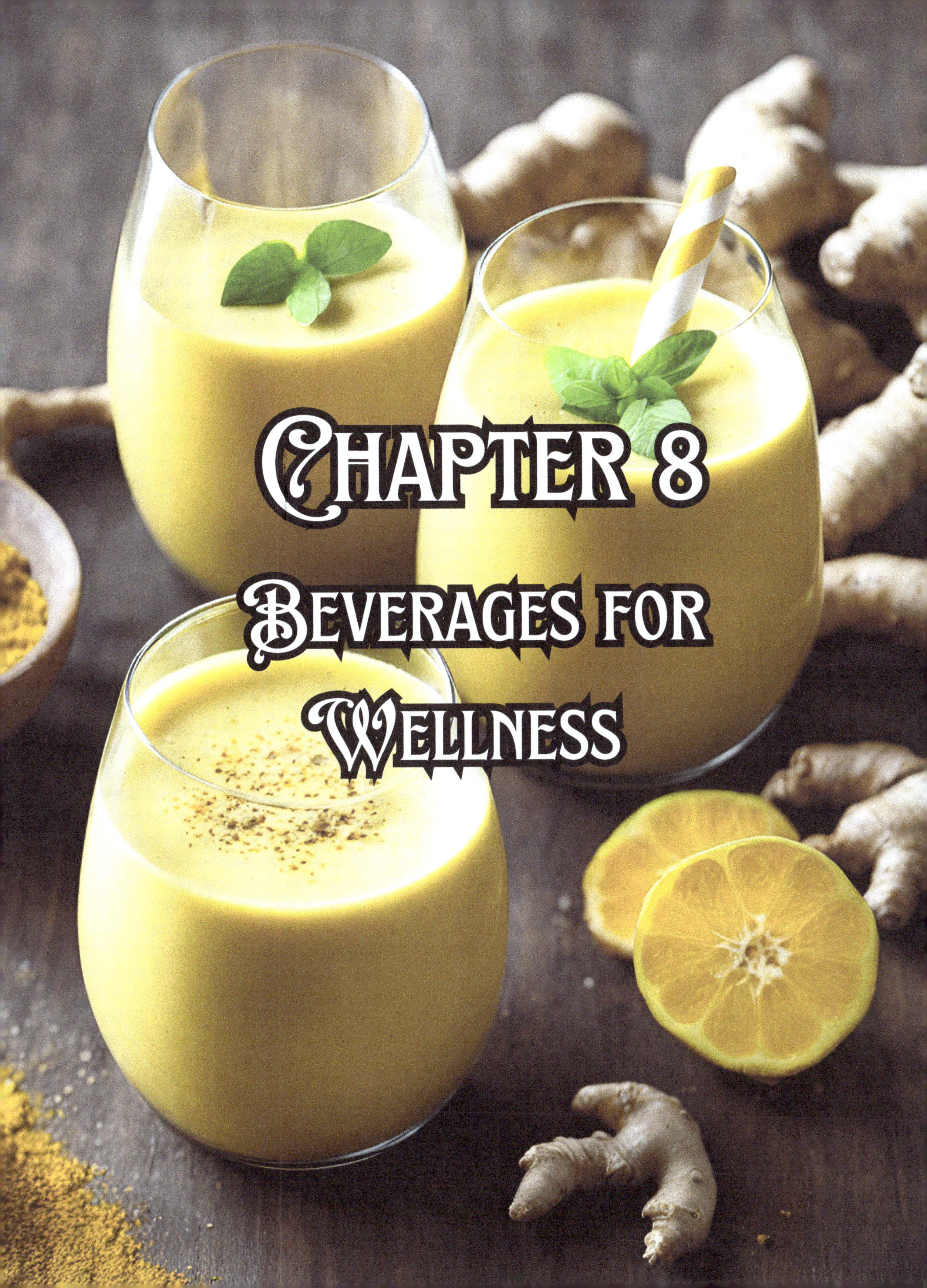
Chapter 8
Beverages for Wellness

WATERMELON COOLER

Ingredients

- 2 cups of diced seedless watermelon
- 1/2 cup of fresh lime juice
- 1 tablespoon of honey or agave syrup (optional)
- Ice cubes
- Fresh mint leaves for garnish (optional)

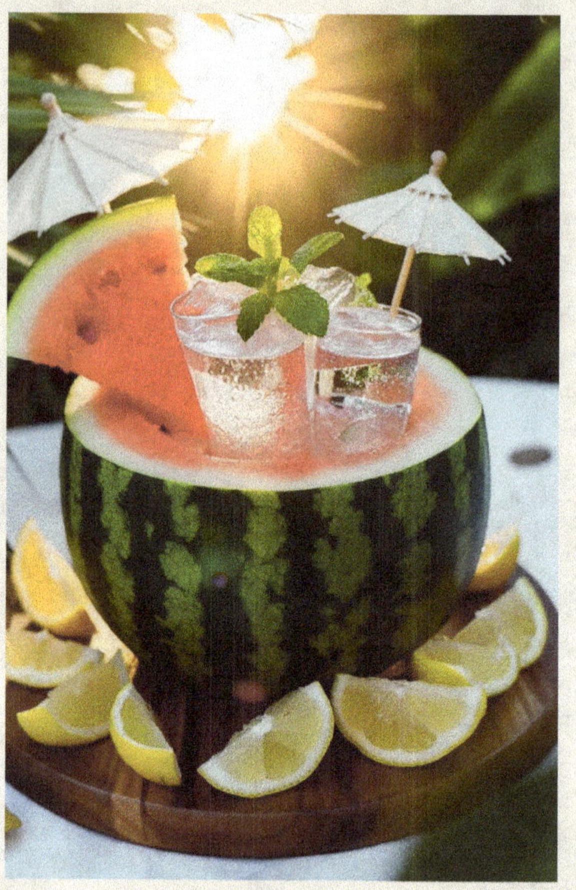

Instructions

- In a blender, combine the diced watermelon, lime juice, and honey (if using).
- Blend until smooth and well combined.
- Taste and adjust sweetness if necessary by adding more honey.
- Fill a glass with ice cubes.
- Pour the watermelon mixture over the ice cubes.
- Garnish with fresh mint leaves if desired.
- Serve immediately and enjoy!

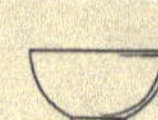 **Preparation Time : 5 min**

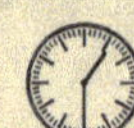 **Total Time : 10 min**

 **Servings : 1**

Nutritional Info

- Calories: 70 kcal
- Total Fat: 0 g
- Saturated Fat: 0 g
- Cholesterol: 0 mg
- Sodium: 2 mg
- Total Carbohydrates: 18 g

CUCUMBER MINT WATER

Ingredients

- 1 medium cucumber, thinly sliced
- 1/4 cup fresh mint leaves
- 1 lemon, thinly sliced
- 4 cups cold water
- Ice cubes (optional)

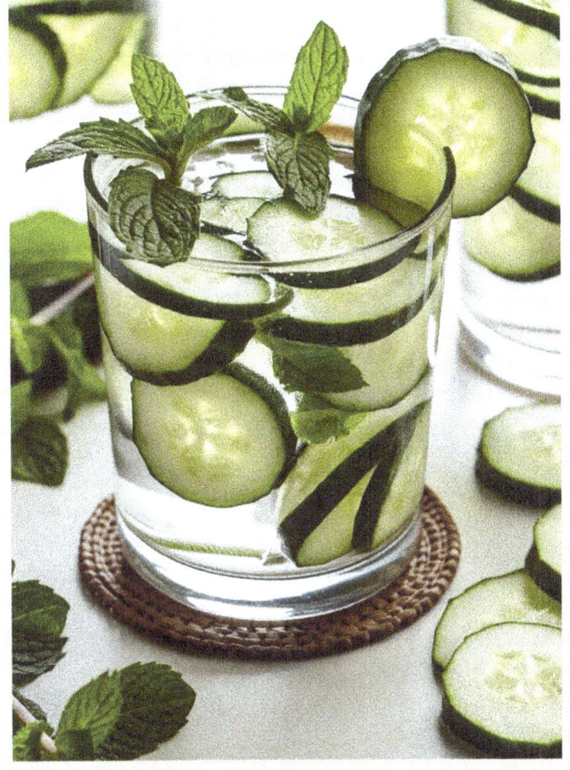

Instructions

- In a large pitcher, add the sliced cucumber, fresh mint leaves, and lemon slices.
- Pour cold water over the ingredients in the pitcher.
- Stir gently to combine.
- Refrigerate the cucumber mint water for at least 1 hour to allow the flavors to infuse.
- Serve chilled over ice cubes, if desired.

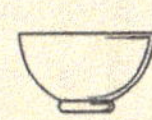 **Preparation Time : 5 min**

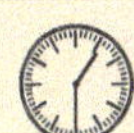 **Total Time : 5 min**

 **Servings : 4**

Nutritional Info

- Calories: 4
- Total Fat: 0g
- Cholesterol: 0mg
- Sodium: 2mg
- Total Carbohydrates: 1g
- Dietary Fiber: 0g

LEMON LIME INFUSION

Ingredients

- 1 lemon, thinly sliced
- 1 lime, thinly sliced
- Ice cubes (optional)
- Water

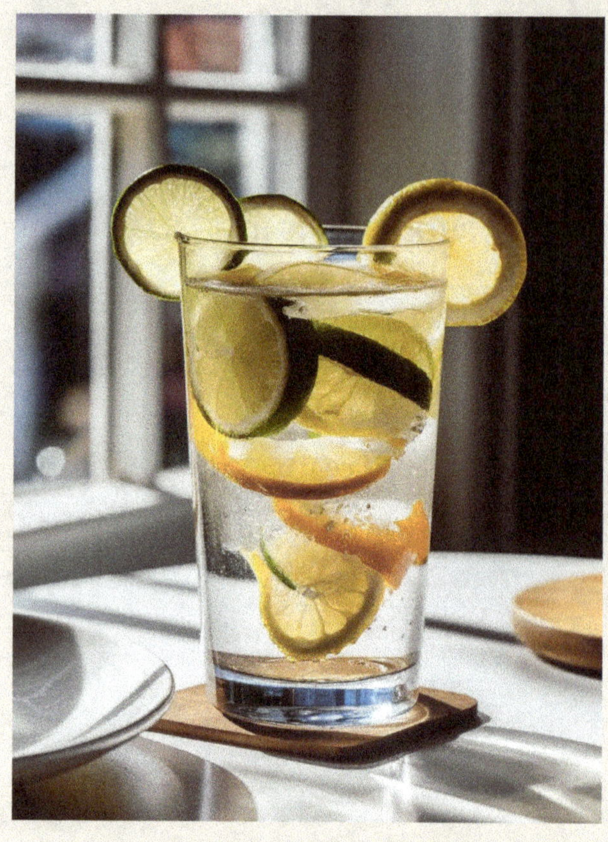

Instructions

- Place lemon and lime slices into a pitcher.
- Add ice cubes if desired.
- Fill the pitcher with water.
- Allow the water to infuse for at least 30 minutes before serving.
- Serve chilled and enjoy!

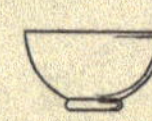 **Preparation Time : 5 min**

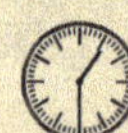 **Total Time : 5 min**

 **Servings : 1**

Nutritional Info

- Calories: 0
- Carbohydrates: 0g
- Fat: 0g
- Protein: 0g

TROPICAL FRUIT SMOOTHIE

Ingredients

- 1/2 cup frozen pineapple chunks
- 1/2 cup frozen mango chunks
- 1/2 cup frozen banana slices
- 1/2 cup coconut water
- 1/4 cup Greek yogurt
- 1 tablespoon honey (optional)
- Juice of 1/2 lime

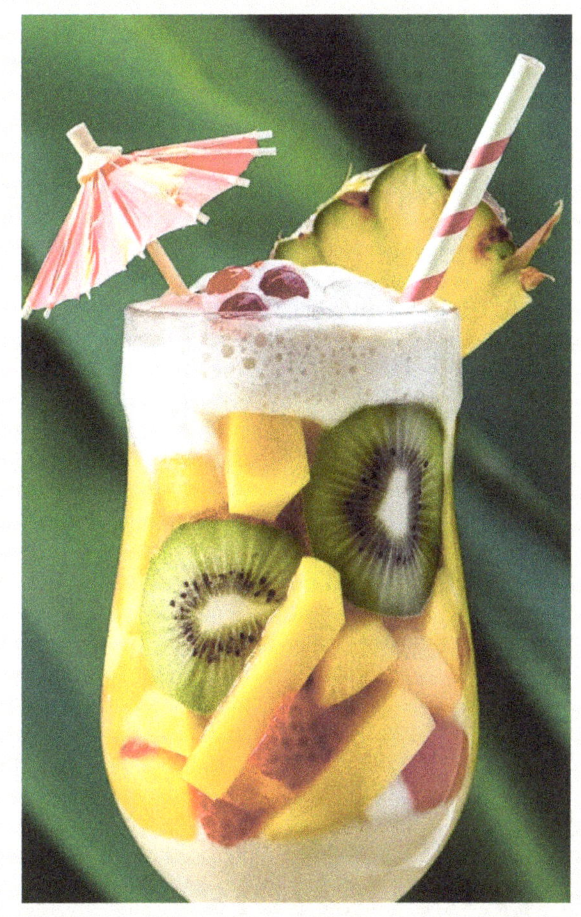

Instructions

- Place the frozen pineapple, mango, and banana chunks in a blender.
- Add the coconut water, Greek yogurt, honey (if using), and lime juice.
- Blend on high speed until smooth and creamy, adding more coconut water if necessary to reach your desired consistency.
- Pour into a glass and serve immediately.

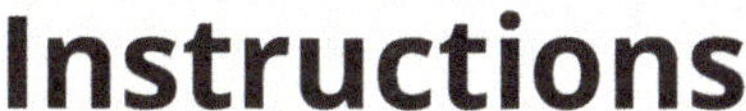 **Preparation Time : 5 min**

Total Time : 5 min

 **Servings : 1**

Nutritional Info

- Calories: 150
- Protein: 3g
- Carbohydrates: 35g
- Fat: 1g
- Fiber: 5g
- Sugar: 25g

BERRY PROTEIN SHAKE

Ingredients

- 1/2 cup mixed berries (strawberries, blueberries, raspberries)
- 1/2 cup unsweetened almond milk
- 1 scoop (about 30g) vanilla protein powder
- 1/4 cup plain Greek yogurt
- 1/2 banana, frozen
- 1/2 cup ice cubes

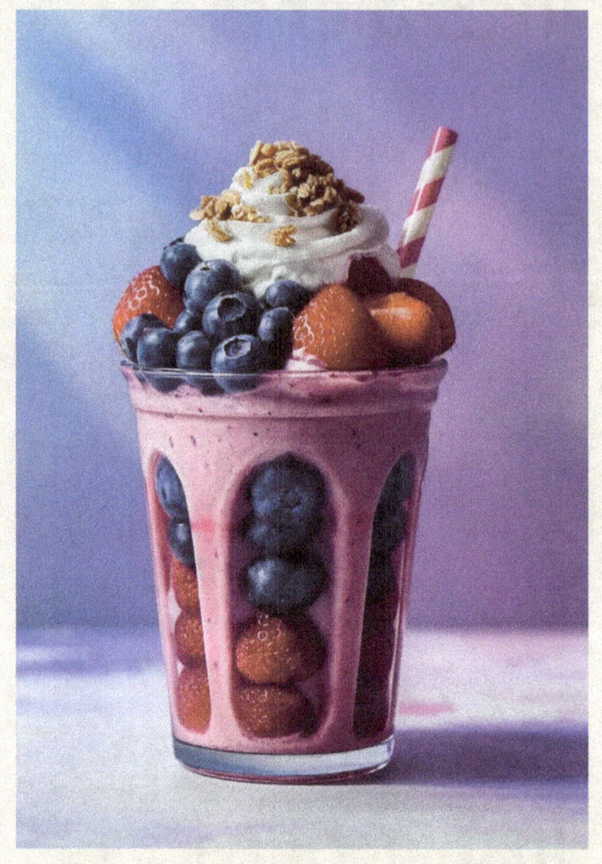

Instructions

- Add all ingredients to a blender.
- Blend on high speed until smooth and creamy, about 1-2 minutes.
- If the shake is too thick, add more almond milk, a little at a time, until desired consistency is reached.
- Pour into a glass and enjoy immediately!

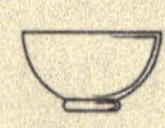 **Preparation Time : 5 min**

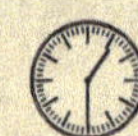 **Total Time : 5 min**

 **Servings : 1**

Nutritional Info

- Calories: 200 kcal
- Protein: 20g
- Carbohydrates: 25g
- Fat: 2g
- Fiber: 5g

SPICED APPLE CIDER

Ingredients

- 6 medium apples, quartered (use a mix of sweet and tart varieties)
- 1 orange, sliced
- 3 cinnamon sticks
- 1 tablespoon whole cloves
- 1 tablespoon whole allspice berries
- 1 teaspoon ground nutmeg
- 8 cups water

Instructions

- In a large pot, combine the quartered apples, orange slices, cinnamon sticks, whole cloves, whole allspice berries, ground nutmeg, and water.
- Bring the mixture to a boil over medium-high heat.
- Once boiling, reduce the heat to low and let the cider simmer for 30 minutes, uncovered, stirring occasionally.
- After 30 minutes, remove the pot from the heat and let it cool slightly.
- Using a fine mesh strainer or cheesecloth, strain the cider into a pitcher or another container to remove the solids.
- Serve the spiced apple cider warm, or refrigerate it for a few hours to serve chilled.
- Optionally, garnish each serving with a cinnamon stick or a slice of fresh apple.

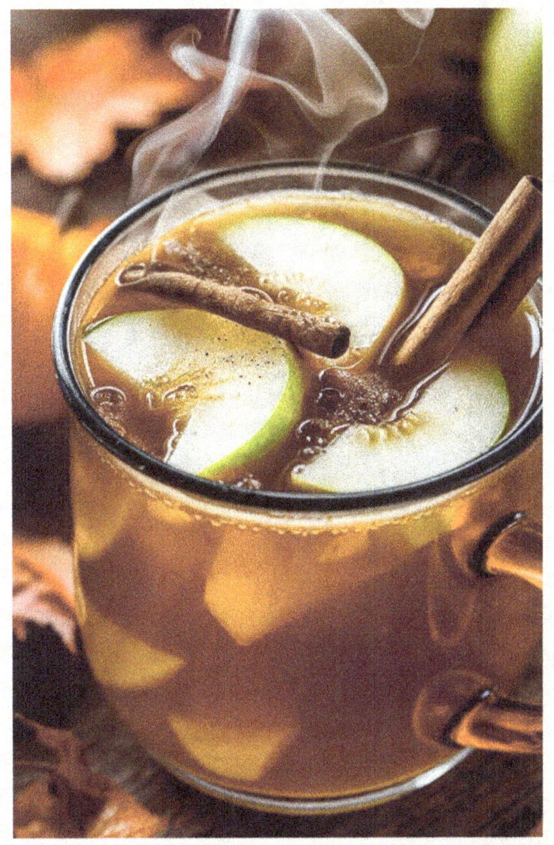

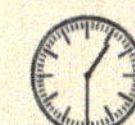 **Preparation Time : 5 min**

 **Total Time : 35 min**

Servings : 4

Nutritional Info

- Calories: 60
- Total Fat: 0g
- Saturated Fat: 0g
- Cholesterol: 0mg
- Sodium: 5mg
- Total Carbohydrates: 16g

MATCHA GREEN TEA LATTE

Ingredients

- 1 teaspoon matcha green tea powder
- 1/4 cup hot water (not boiling)
- 3/4 cup unsweetened almond milk (or any milk of choice)
- 1-2 teaspoons honey or sweetener of choice (optional)

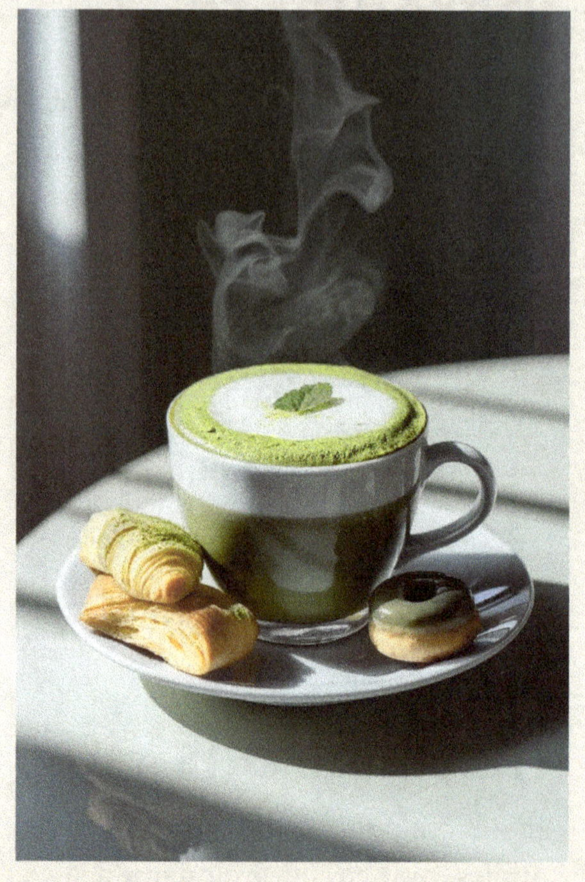

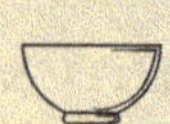 **Preparation Time : 5 min**

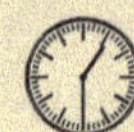 **Total Time : 10 min**

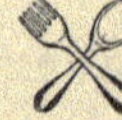 **Servings : 1**

Instructions

- Prepare Matcha: Sift 1 teaspoon of matcha green tea powder into a mug to avoid clumps.
- Add Water: Pour 1/4 cup of hot water (not boiling) into the mug with the matcha powder. Whisk vigorously using a bamboo whisk or a small regular whisk until the matcha is fully dissolved and frothy.
- Heat Milk: In a small saucepan, heat 3/4 cup of unsweetened almond milk over medium heat until it is warm but not boiling. You can also heat the milk in the microwave for about 1-2 minutes.
- Combine: Pour the heated milk into the mug with the matcha mixture. Stir to combine.
- Sweeten (Optional): If desired, add 1-2 teaspoons of honey or your preferred sweetener and stir until dissolved.
- Serve: Enjoy your Matcha Green Tea Latte immediately while warm.

Nutritional Info

- Calories: 40 (without sweetener)
- Protein: 1g
- Fat: 3g
- Carbohydrates: 2g
- Fiber: 1g
- Sugar: 0g (without sweetener)

GREEN DETOX SMOOTHIE

Ingredients

- 1 cup spinach, washed
- 1/2 cup kale, washed and stems removed
- 1/2 ripe avocado, peeled and pitted
- 1/2 banana, peeled
- 1/2 cup cucumber, peeled and chopped
- 1/2 cup unsweetened almond milk (or any milk of choice)
- Juice of 1/2 lemon
- 1 teaspoon grated ginger

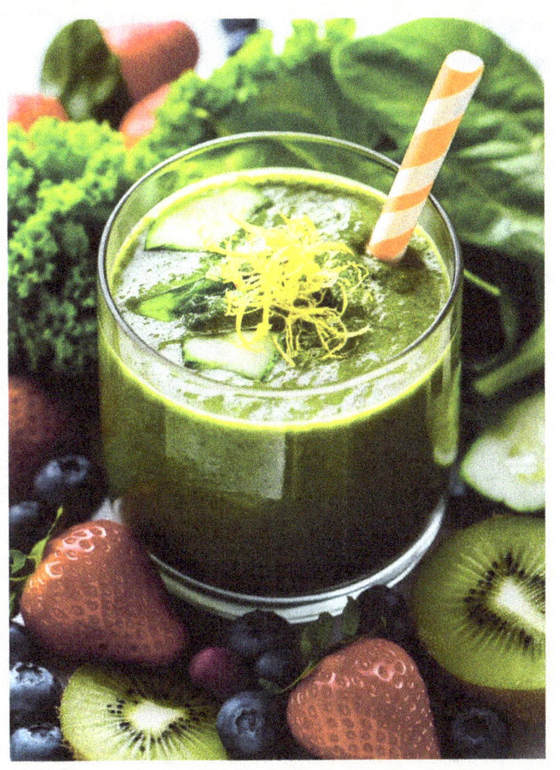

Instructions

- Place all the ingredients into a blender.
- Blend on high speed until smooth and creamy.
- If the smoothie is too thick, add more almond milk to reach your desired consistency.
- Taste and adjust sweetness by adding more banana if needed.
- Pour into a glass and enjoy immediately.

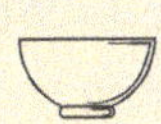 **Preparation Time : 5 min**

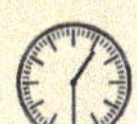 **Total Time : 5 min**

 **Servings : 1**

Nutritional Info

- Calories: 150 kcal
- Protein: 5g
- Carbohydrates: 25g
- Fat: 3g
- Fiber: 8g

HERBAL ICED TEA

Ingredients

- 1 herbal tea bag (such as chamomile, peppermint, or hibiscus)
- 1 cup water
- Ice cubes
- Optional: sweetener of your choice (honey, stevia, agave syrup)

Instructions

- Boil 1 cup of water in a kettle or saucepan.
- Place the herbal tea bag in a heat-proof glass or mug.
- Pour the boiling water over the tea bag.
- Let the tea steep for 3-5 minutes, depending on your desired strength.
- Remove the tea bag and discard it.
- Allow the brewed tea to cool to room temperature.
- Once cooled, transfer the tea to a glass filled with ice cubes.
- Optionally, sweeten the tea with your preferred sweetener, stirring until dissolved.
- Garnish with a slice of lemon, a sprig of mint, or a slice of cucumber, if desired.
- Serve immediately and enjoy your refreshing Herbal Iced Tea!

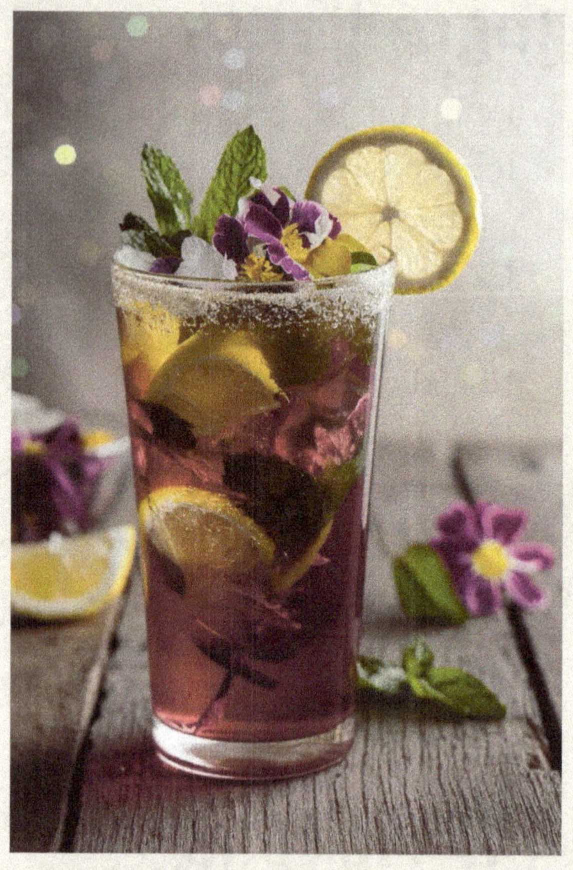

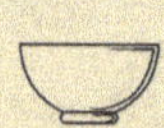 **Preparation Time : 5 min**

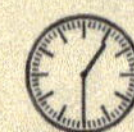 **Total Time : 5 min**

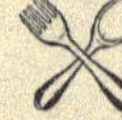 **Servings : 1**

Nutritional Info

- Calories: 0 kcal
- Carbohydrates: 0 g
- Protein: 0 g
- Fat: 0 g
- Fiber: 0 g

BERRY LEMONADE

Ingredients

- 1 cup fresh strawberries, hulled and sliced
- 1 cup fresh blueberries
- 1 cup fresh raspberries
- 1 cup fresh blackberries
- 1 cup fresh lemon juice (about 4-6 lemons)
- 4 cups cold water
- 1-2 tablespoons honey or a natural sweetener (optional)
- Ice cubes
- Fresh mint leaves for garnish (optional)

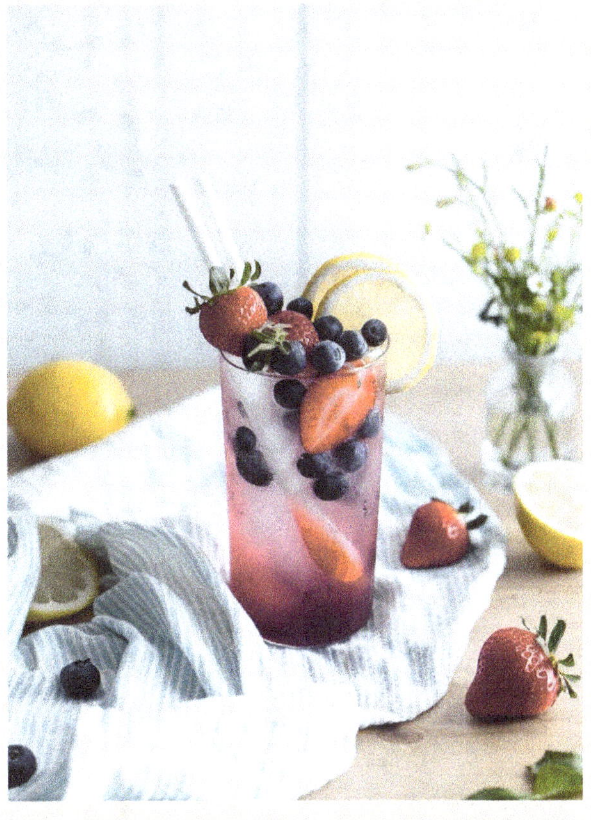

Instructions

- Wash the strawberries, blueberries, raspberries, and blackberries thoroughly.
- Hull and slice the strawberries.
- Place the strawberries, blueberries, raspberries, and blackberries in a blender.
- Blend until smooth.
- Pour the blended berry mixture through a fine mesh sieve or cheesecloth into a large pitcher to remove seeds and pulp. Use a spoon to press the mixture through the sieve if needed.
- Add the freshly squeezed lemon juice to the pitcher.
- Pour in the cold water and stir well.
- If desired, add honey or your preferred natural sweetener to the pitcher and stir until dissolved.
- Fill glasses with ice cubes.
- Pour the berry lemonade over the ice.
- Garnish with fresh mint leaves if desired.
- Serve immediately and enjoy your refreshing berry lemonade!

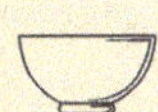 **Preparation Time : 15 min**

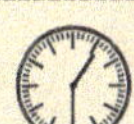 **Total Time : 15 min**

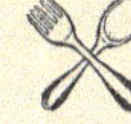 **Servings : 4**

Nutritional Info

- Calories: 50
- Protein: 1g
- Carbohydrates: 13g
- Dietary Fiber: 4g
- Sugars: 9g
- Fat: 0g

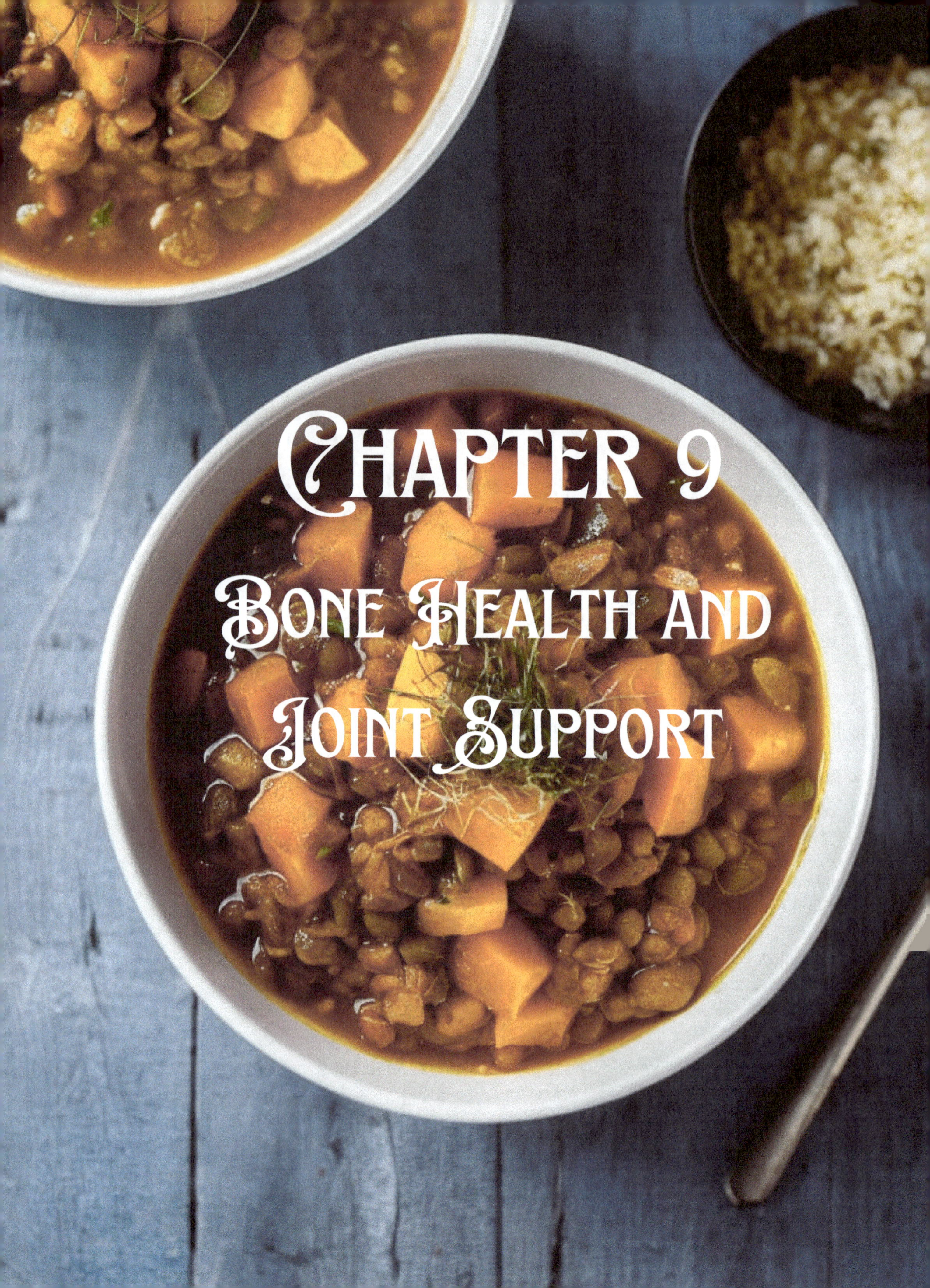

Chapter 9
Bone Health and
Joint Support

SARDINE AND ARUGULA SALAD

Ingredients

- 2 cans of sardines, drained
- 4 cups fresh arugula
- 1 cup cherry tomatoes, halved
- 1/4 red onion, thinly sliced
- 1/4 cup Kalamata olives, pitted
- 2 tablespoons extra virgin olive oil
- 1 tablespoon balsamic vinegar
- Salt and pepper to taste

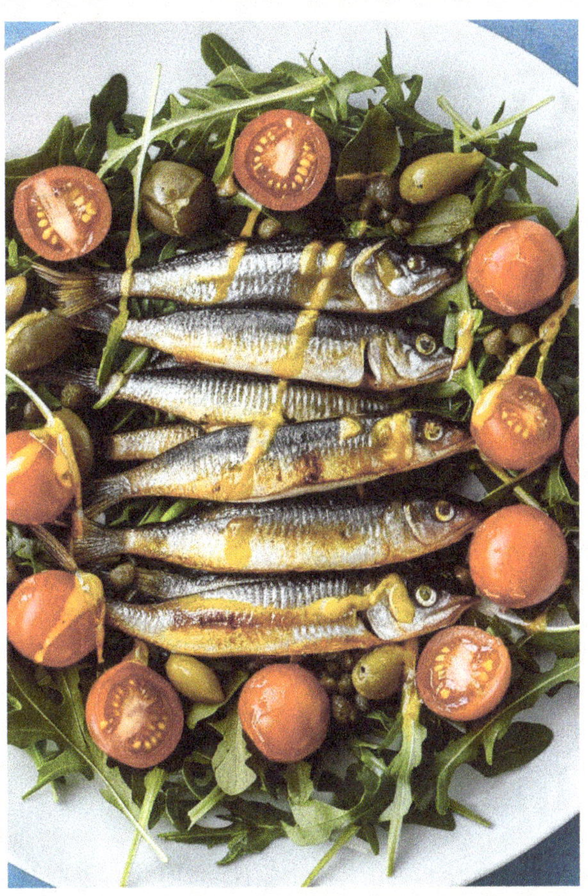

Instructions

- In a large bowl, combine the arugula, cherry tomatoes, red onion, and Kalamata olives.
- Add the drained sardines on top.
- In a small bowl, whisk together the olive oil, balsamic vinegar, salt, and pepper.
- Drizzle the dressing over the salad and gently toss to combine.
- Serve immediately.

Preparation Time : 10 min

Total Time : 10 min

Servings : 2

Nutritional Info

- Calories: 320 kcal
- Protein: 24g
- Carbohydrates: 7g
- Fat: 22g
- Fiber: 2g

ALMOND-CRUSTED CHICKEN TENDERS

Ingredients

- 1 lb chicken tenders
- 1 cup almond flour
- 2 eggs, beaten
- 1 tsp garlic powder
- 1 tsp paprika
- Salt and pepper to taste
- Cooking spray or olive oil

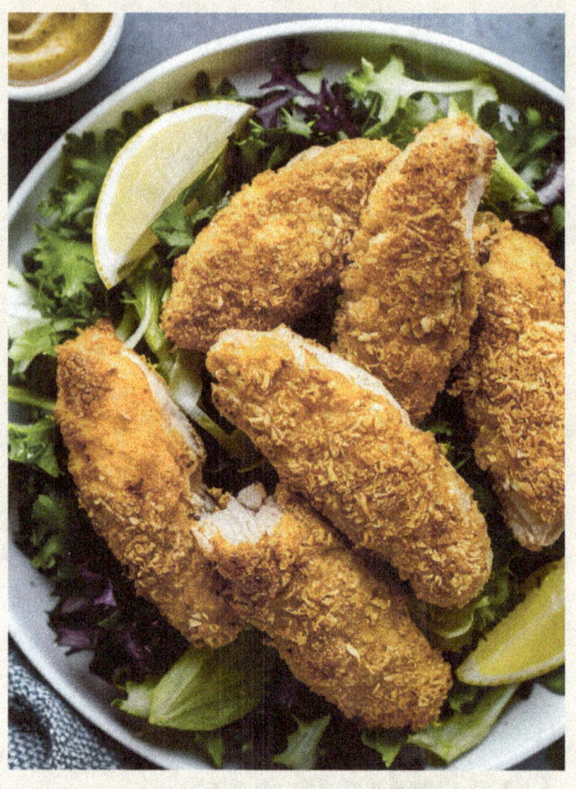

Instructions

- Preheat your oven to 400°F (200°C).
- In a shallow dish, mix almond flour, garlic powder, paprika, salt, and pepper.
- Dip each chicken tender into the beaten eggs, then coat with the almond flour mixture, pressing gently to adhere.
- Place the coated tenders on a baking sheet lined with parchment paper or aluminum foil.
- Lightly spray or drizzle with olive oil.
- Bake for 15-20 minutes or until the chicken is cooked through and the coating is golden brown and crispy.
- Serve hot with your favorite dipping sauce.

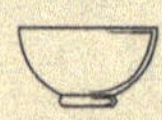 **Preparation Time : 10 min**

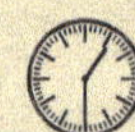 **Total Time : 25 min**

 **Servings : 4**

Nutritional Info

- Calories: 290 kcal
- Protein: 30g
- Fat: 16g
- Saturated Fat: 2g
- Trans Fat: 0g

BROCCOLI AND KALE SOUP

Ingredients

- 2 cups broccoli florets
- 1 cup chopped kale leaves
- 1 onion, diced
- 2 cloves garlic, minced
- 4 cups vegetable broth
- 1 tablespoon olive oil
- Salt and pepper to taste

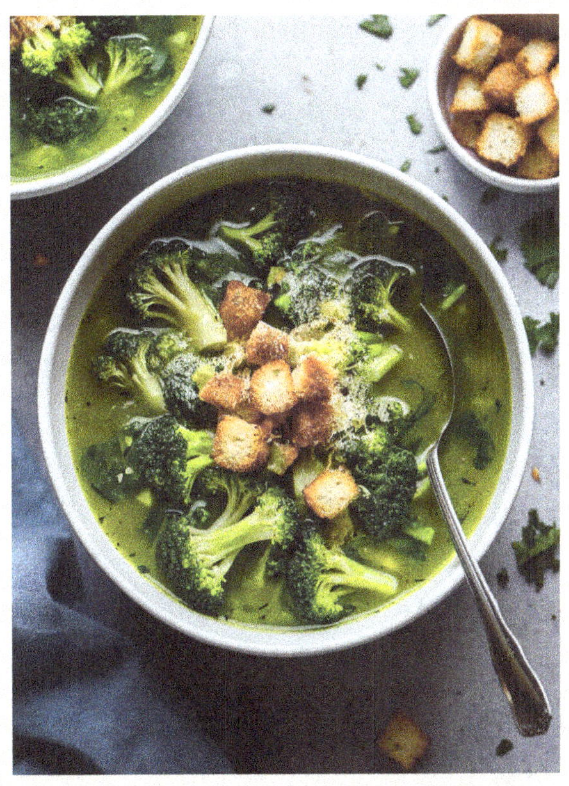

Instructions

- Heat olive oil in a large pot over medium heat. Add diced onion and minced garlic, sauté until fragrant.
- Add broccoli florets and chopped kale leaves to the pot. Cook for 5 minutes, stirring occasionally.
- Pour vegetable broth into the pot. Bring to a boil, then reduce heat and simmer for 15-20 minutes until vegetables are tender.
- Use an immersion blender or transfer soup to a blender to puree until smooth.
- Season with salt and pepper to taste. If desired, add red pepper flakes for heat.
- Serve hot, garnished with grated Parmesan if desired.

Preparation Time : 10 min

Total Time : 30 min

Servings : 4

Nutritional Info

- Calories: 120 kcal
- Protein: 4g
- Carbohydrates: 15g
- Fat: 6g
- Fiber: 5g

SESAME GINGER TOFU

Ingredients

- 1 block (14 oz) firm tofu, drained and pressed
- 2 tbsp soy sauce
- 1 tbsp sesame oil
- 1 tbsp rice vinegar
- 1 tbsp maple syrup or honey
- 2 cloves garlic, minced
- 1 tbsp freshly grated ginger or ginger paste
- 2 tbsp sesame seeds
- 2 green onions, thinly sliced
- 1 tbsp cornstarch
- 2 tbsp water

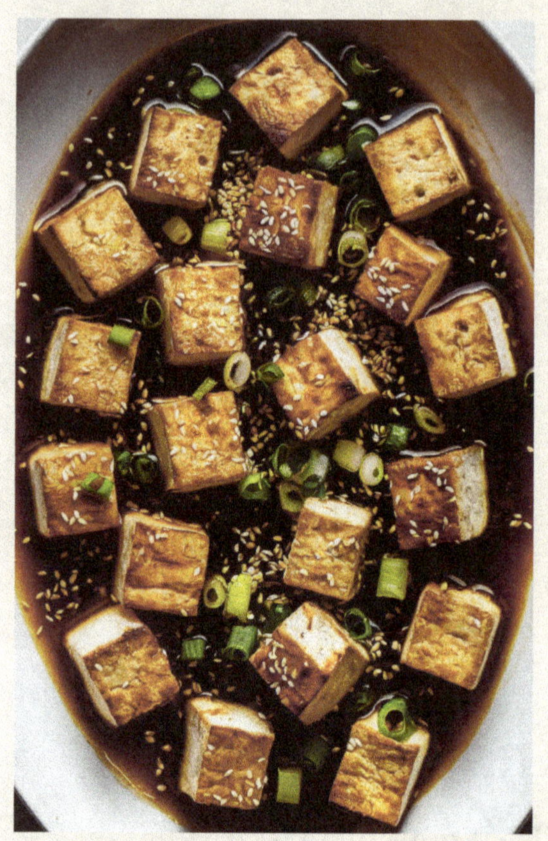

Instructions

- Cut tofu into cubes or slices.
- In a bowl, mix soy sauce, sesame oil, rice vinegar, maple syrup, minced garlic, grated ginger, and sesame seeds.
- Toss tofu in the marinade, coat evenly.
- Let it sit for 15-30 minutes.
- Mix cornstarch and water in a small bowl.
- Heat cooking oil in a pan over medium-high heat.
- Dip each tofu piece in the cornstarch mixture.
- Fry tofu until golden brown and crispy, about 3-4 minutes per side.
- Remove from pan and drain excess oil on paper towels.
- Garnish with sliced green onions and sesame seeds.
- Serve hot as a main dish or with rice and vegetables.

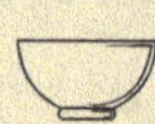 **Preparation Time : 15 min**

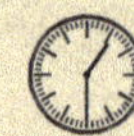 **Total Time : 25 min**

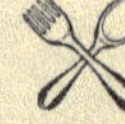 **Servings : 4**

Nutritional Info

- Calories: 220 kcal
- Protein: 14g
- Carbohydrates: 10g
- Fat: 15g
- Fiber: 2g

CITRUS AND WALNUT SALAD

Ingredients

- 4 cups mixed salad greens
- 1 orange, segmented
- 1 grapefruit, segmented
- ½ cup walnuts, toasted
- ¼ cup crumbled feta cheese (optional)
- 2 tablespoons extra virgin olive oil
- 1 tablespoon balsamic vinegar
- Salt and pepper to taste

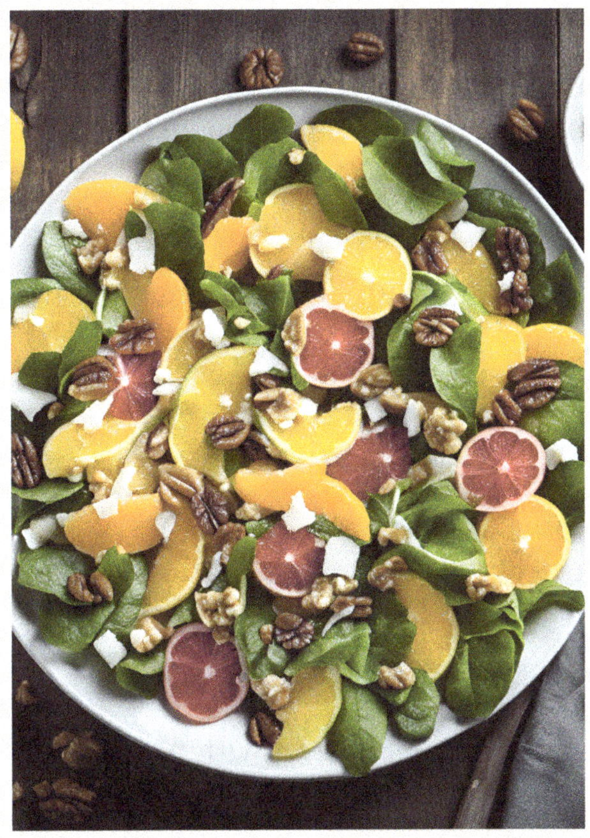

Instructions

- In a large bowl, combine the mixed salad greens, orange segments, and grapefruit segments.
- In a dry skillet over medium heat, toast the walnuts for 2-3 minutes until fragrant, then remove from heat and let them cool.
- Add the toasted walnuts to the bowl with the salad greens and citrus segments.
- If using, sprinkle the crumbled feta cheese over the salad.
- In a small bowl, whisk together the extra virgin olive oil and balsamic vinegar to make the dressing.
- Drizzle the dressing over the salad and toss gently to coat.
- Season with salt and pepper to taste.
- Serve immediately.

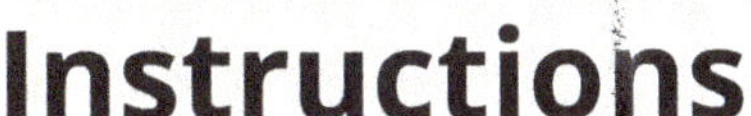

Preparation Time : 10 min

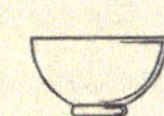

Total Time : 15 min

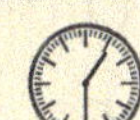

Servings : 4

Nutritional Info

- Calories: 210 kcal
- Total Fat: 18g
- Saturated Fat: 2g
- Trans Fat: 0g
- Cholesterol: 0mg
- Sodium: 90mg

SPINACH AND RICOTTA STUFFED PORTOBELLOS

Ingredients

- 4 large portobello mushrooms
- 2 cups fresh spinach, chopped
- 1 cup ricotta cheese
- 1/2 cup grated Parmesan cheese
- 2 cloves garlic, minced
- Salt and pepper to taste
- Olive oil for drizzling

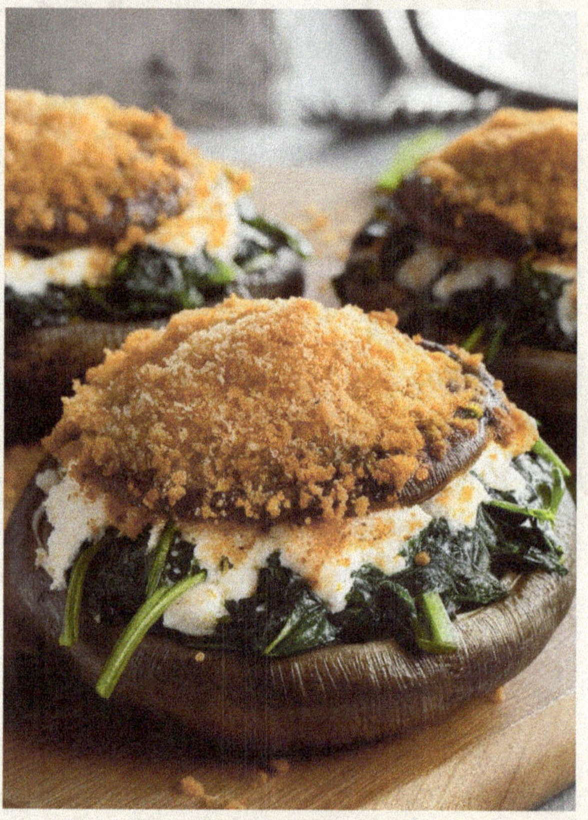

Instructions

- Preheat the oven to 375°F (190°C). Line a baking sheet with parchment paper.
- Clean the portobello mushrooms and remove the stems. Place them on the prepared baking sheet, gill side up.
- In a mixing bowl, combine chopped spinach, ricotta cheese, Parmesan cheese, minced garlic, salt, and pepper. Mix well.
- Spoon the spinach and ricotta mixture evenly into each portobello mushroom cap, filling them to the top.
- Drizzle olive oil over the stuffed mushrooms.
- Bake in the preheated oven for 20-25 minutes, or until the mushrooms are tender and the filling is golden brown.
- Garnish with fresh basil leaves if desired before serving.

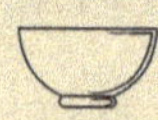 **Preparation Time : 15 min**

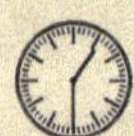 **Total Time : 40 min**

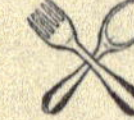 **Servings : 4**

Nutritional Info

- Calories: 185 kcal
- Protein: 12g
- Carbohydrates: 8g
- Fat: 12g
- Fiber: 2g

MISO SOUP WITH SEAWEED

Ingredients

- 4 cups water
- 4 tablespoons miso paste
- 1 sheet nori seaweed, shredded
- 1 cup firm tofu, cubed
- 2 green onions, thinly sliced
- Optional: 1 tablespoon soy sauce or tamari for extra flavor

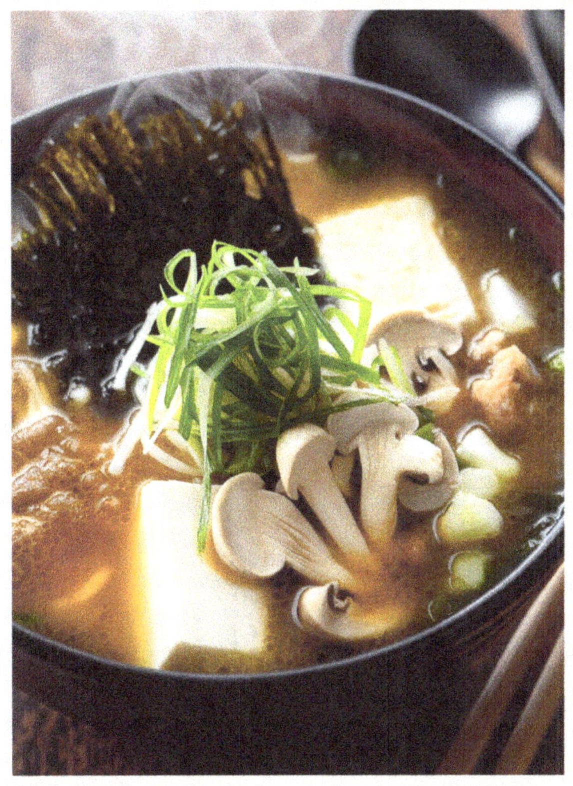

Instructions

- In a pot, bring water to a gentle boil.
- Reduce heat to low and whisk in miso paste until dissolved.
- Add shredded nori and tofu cubes, simmer for 5 minutes.
- Remove from heat and stir in green onions.
- Serve hot and enjoy!

Preparation Time : 10 min

Total Time : 15 min

Servings : 4

Nutritional Info

- Calories: 90
- Total Fat: 4g
- Saturated Fat: 0.5g
- Trans Fat: 0g
- Cholesterol: 0mg

CALCIUM-RICH SMOOTHIE

Ingredients

- 1 cup kale leaves, stemmed
- 1 ripe banana
- 1/2 cup plain Greek yogurt
- 1/2 cup almond milk
- 1 tablespoon almond butter
- 1 tablespoon honey
- Ice cubes (optional)

Instructions

- Place all ingredients into a blender.
- Blend until smooth and creamy.
- If desired, add ice cubes and blend again until desired consistency is reached.
- Pour into glasses and serve immediately.

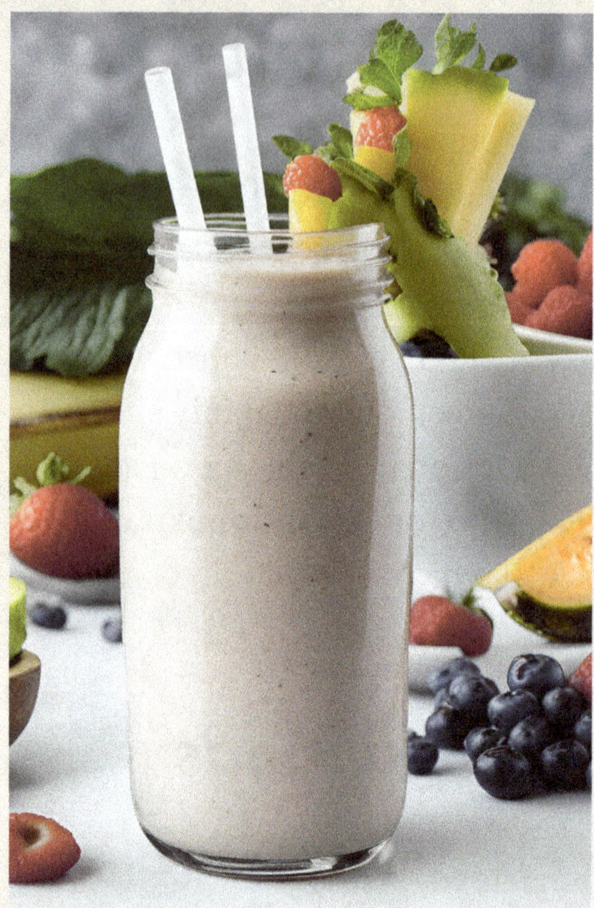

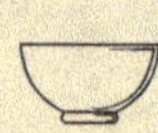
Preparation Time : 5 min

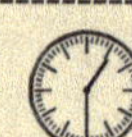
Total Time : 5 min

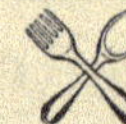
Servings : 2

Nutritional Info

- Calories: 180
- Protein: 9g
- Fat: 5g
- Carbohydrates: 30g
- Calcium: 25%

COLLARD GREEN WRAPS

Ingredients

- Large collard green leaves
- Hummus
- Sliced avocado
- Sliced cucumber
- Shredded carrots
- Sliced bell peppers
- Cooked quinoa or brown rice (optional)
- Sliced tofu or grilled chicken (optional)

Instructions

- Wash the collard green leaves and pat them dry.
- Lay a collard green leaf flat on a clean surface.
- Spread a layer of hummus evenly across the leaf, leaving about an inch of space around the edges.
- Layer on sliced avocado, cucumber, shredded carrots, and bell peppers, along with any optional ingredients like quinoa or tofu/chicken.
- Carefully roll up the collard green leaf, tucking in the sides as you go, to form a wrap.
- Secure the wrap with toothpicks if needed.
- Slice the wrap in half diagonally.
- Serve immediately with your favorite sauce or dressing for dipping.

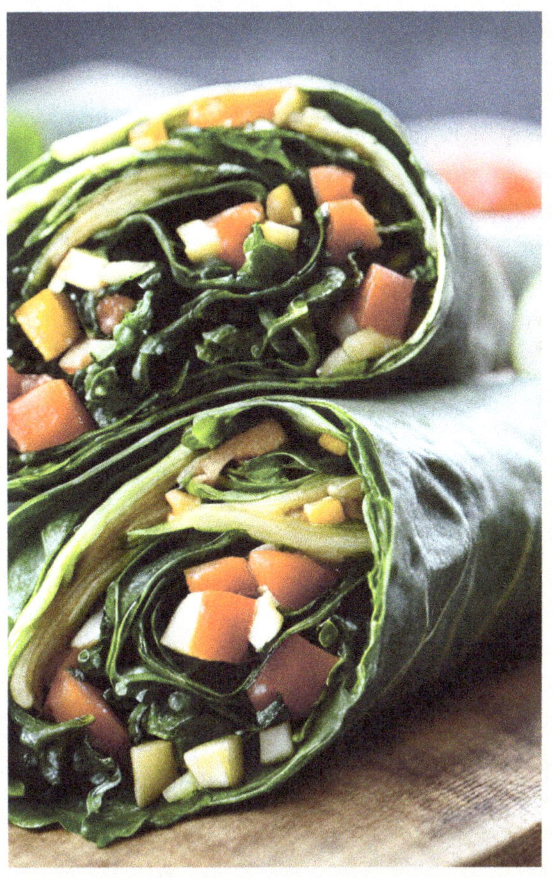

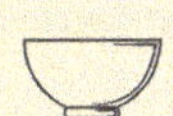 **Preparation Time : 15 min**

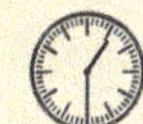 **Total Time : 15 min**

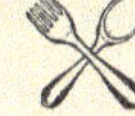 **Servings : 4**

Nutritional Info

- Calories: Approximately 150-200 calories
- Protein: 5-10 grams
- Fat: 8-12 grams
- Carbohydrates: 15-20 grams
- Fiber: 5-8 grams

ORANGE AND ALMOND SALAD

Ingredients

- 2 large oranges, peeled and sliced
- 1/4 cup sliced almonds
- 4 cups mixed salad greens
- 1 tablespoon olive oil
- 1 tablespoon balsamic vinegar
- Salt and pepper to taste

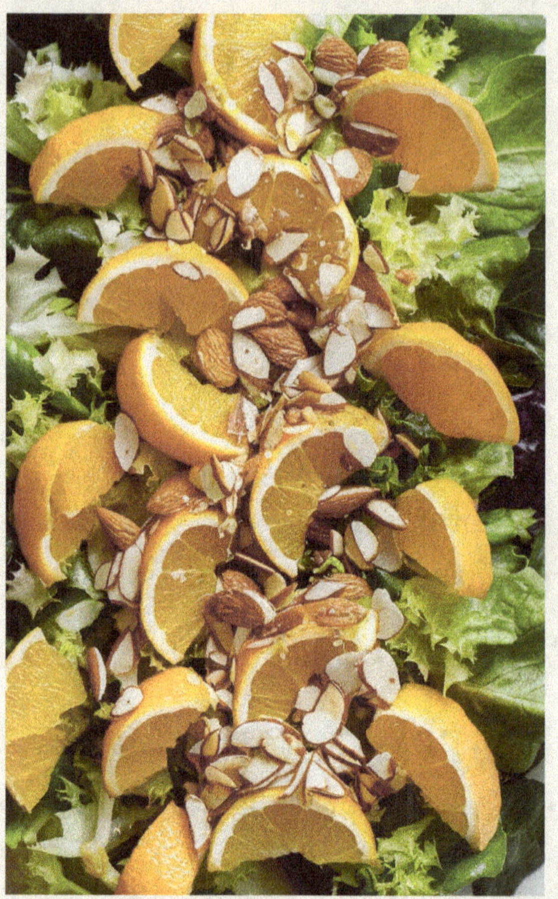

Instructions

- In a dry skillet, toast the sliced almonds over medium heat until golden brown and fragrant, about 3-4 minutes. Remove from heat and set aside.
- In a large bowl, combine the mixed salad greens with the sliced oranges.
- In a small bowl, whisk together the olive oil and balsamic vinegar to make the dressing.
- Drizzle the dressing over the salad and toss gently to coat.
- Sprinkle the toasted almonds over the top of the salad.
- Season with salt and pepper to taste.
- Serve immediately and enjoy!

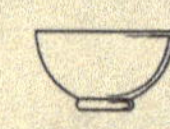 **Preparation Time : 10 min**

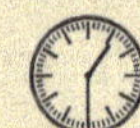 **Total Time : 10 min**

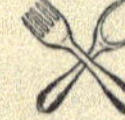 **Servings : 4**

Nutritional Info

- Calories: 120 kcal
- Total Fat: 8g
- Saturated Fat: 1g
- Trans Fat: 0g
- Cholesterol: 0mg
- Sodium: 80mg

CONCLUSION

Thank you for embarking on this culinary journey with us through "Endomorph Diet for Women Over 60." We hope this cookbook has not only provided you with a treasure trove of delicious, nutritious recipes but also empowered you with the knowledge and tools to take control of your health and well-being.

As you turn the last page, take a moment to celebrate your commitment to a healthier lifestyle. The recipes and tips within these pages are designed to nourish your body, satisfy your taste buds, and enhance your life. Each meal you prepare and enjoy is a step toward a stronger, more vibrant you.

The endomorph diet, tailored specifically for women over 60, is more than a diet—it's a lifestyle transformation. It's about understanding your body, fueling it with the right nutrients, and embracing a balanced approach to eating that honors your unique needs. This cookbook is a roadmap to a healthier future, filled with vibrant flavors and wholesome ingredients that support your journey.

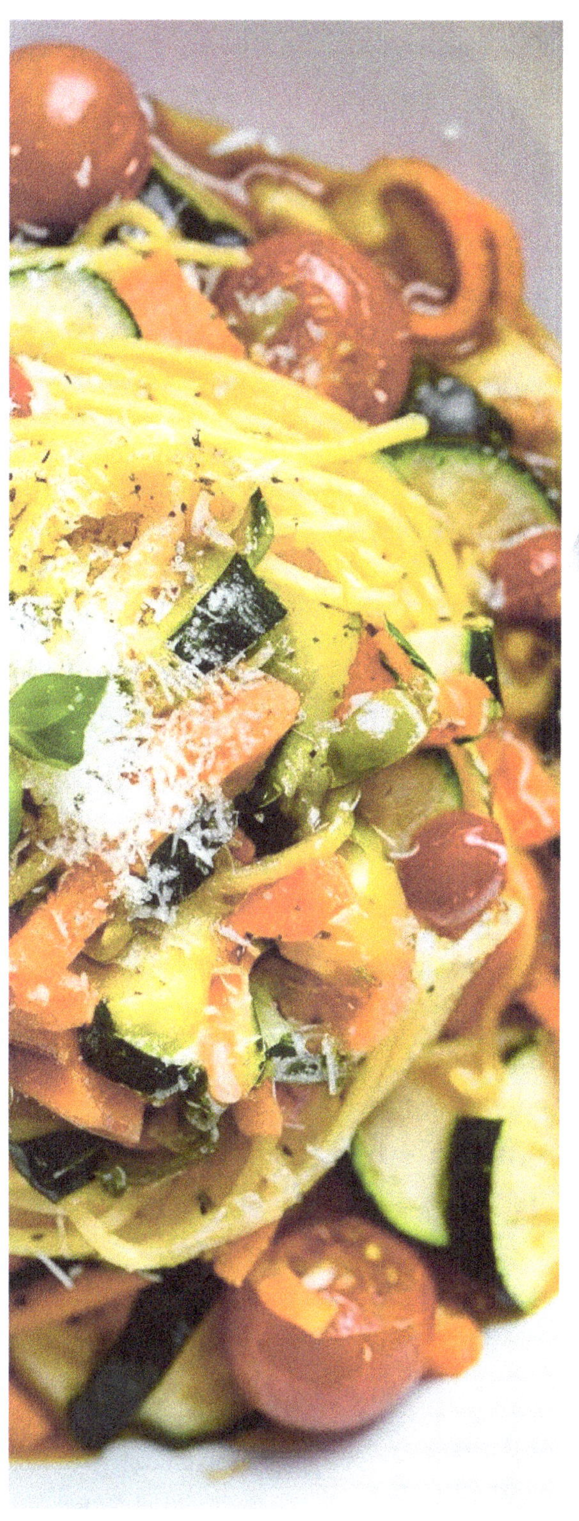

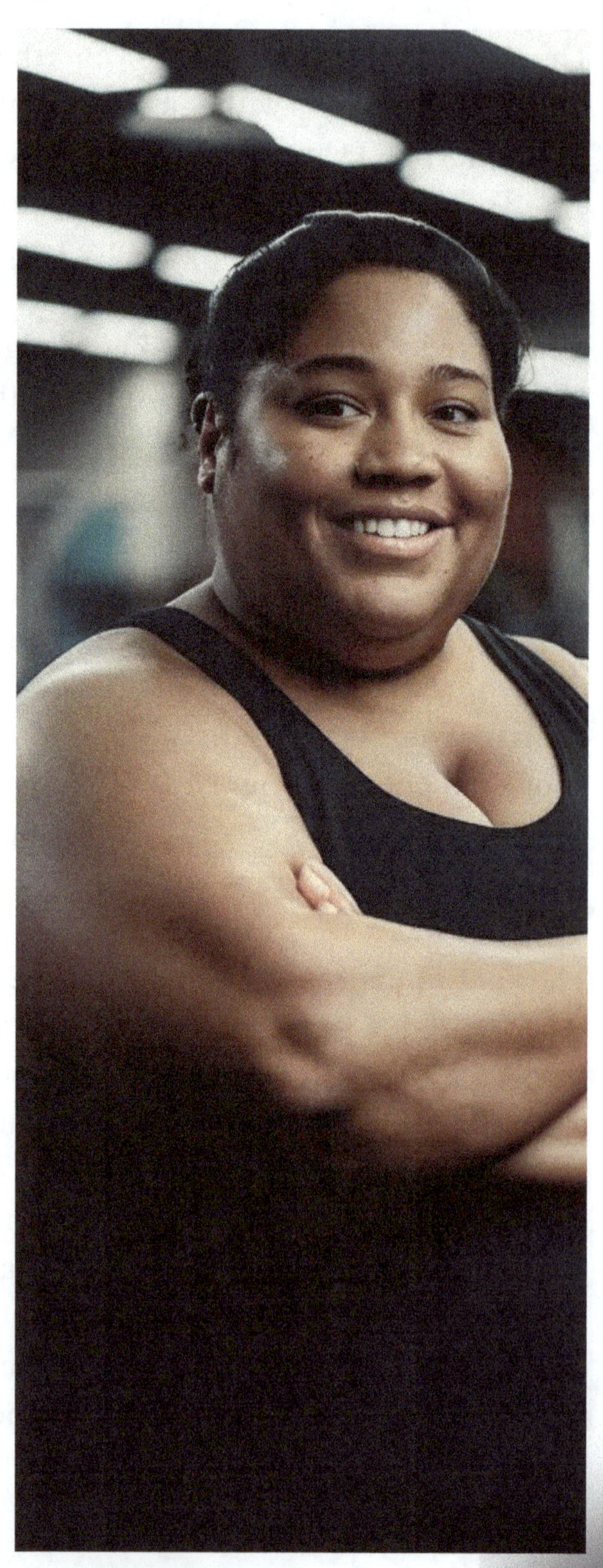

Remember, you are not alone on this journey. Join online communities, seek support from friends and family, and share your successes and challenges. The collective wisdom and encouragement of a supportive community can be a powerful motivator.

As you continue to explore and adapt these recipes to suit your tastes and lifestyle, keep experimenting and discovering new flavors. Let this cookbook be a starting point for your culinary adventures, inspiring you to create meals that are both healthy and delightful.

Here's to the new chapter you've started, one filled with delicious meals, healthier choices, and a renewed sense of well-being. May each recipe bring you joy and satisfaction, and may your journey be as rewarding as the meals you create.

Wishing you endless culinary success and a lifetime of health and happiness. Cheers to you and your vibrant future!

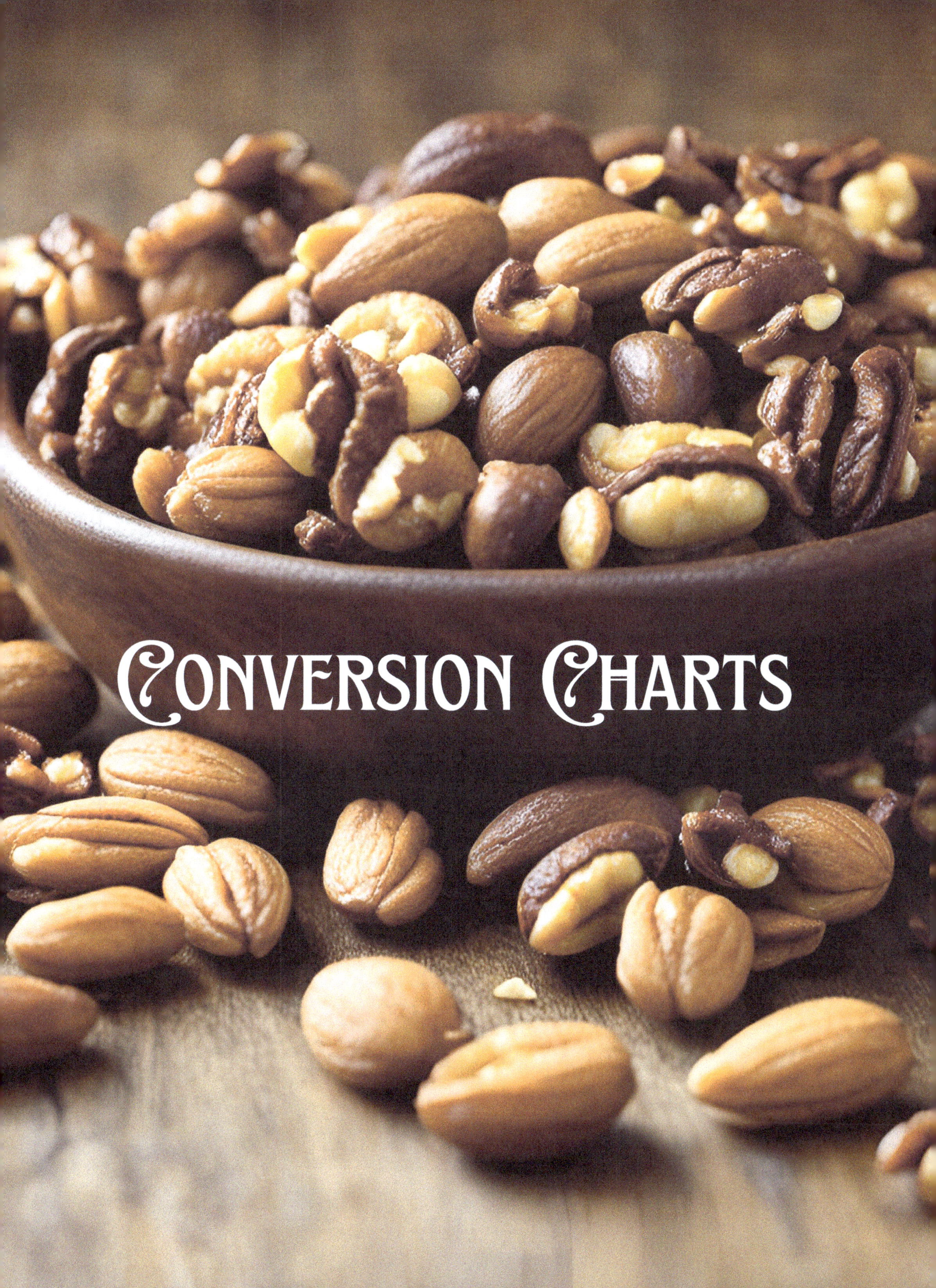

CONVERSION CHARTS

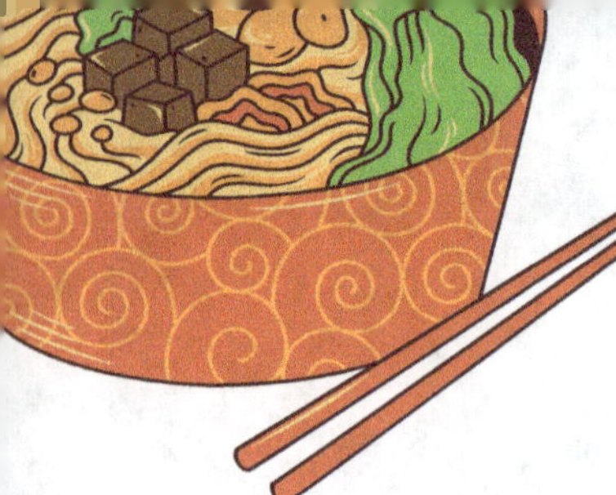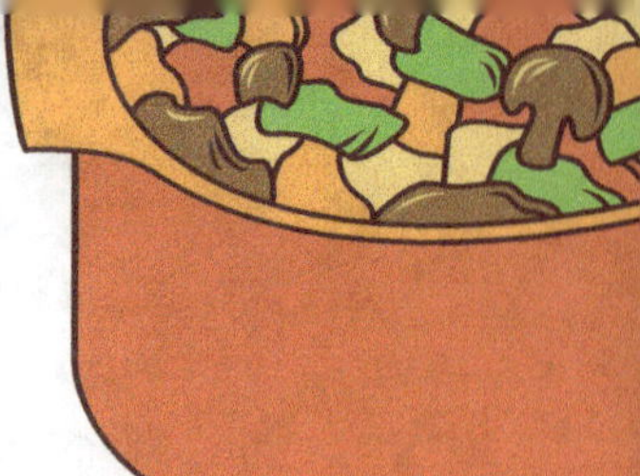

COMMON COOKING MEASUREMENTS

Volume Measurements

MEASUREMENT	EQUIVALENT
1 teaspoon (tsp)	1/3 tablespoon (tbsp)
1 teaspoon (tsp)	3 teaspoons (tsp)
1/8 cup	2 tablespoons (tbsp)
1/4 cup	4 tablespoons (tbsp)
1/3 cup	5 tablespoons + 1 teaspoon
1/2 cup	8 tablespoons (tbsp)
3/4 cup	12 tablespoons (tbsp)
1 cup	16 tablespoons (tbsp)
1 pint (pt)	2 cups
1 quart (qt)	4 cups
1 gallon (gal)	16 cups

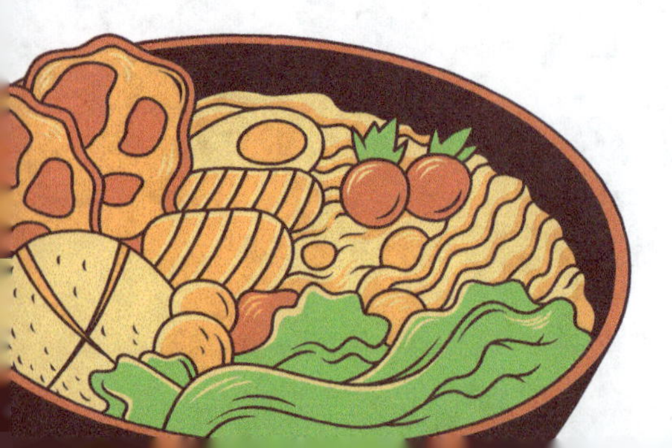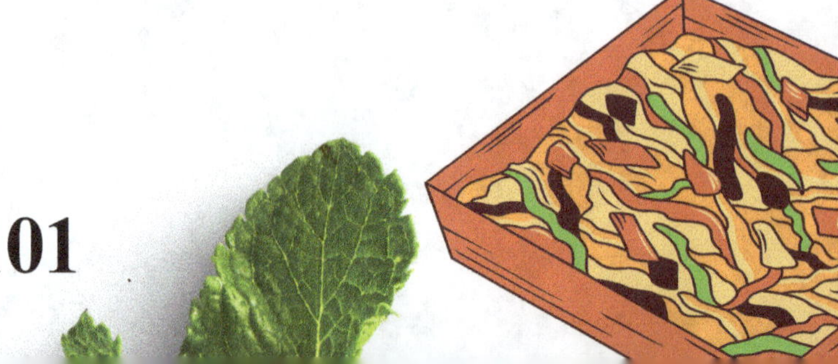

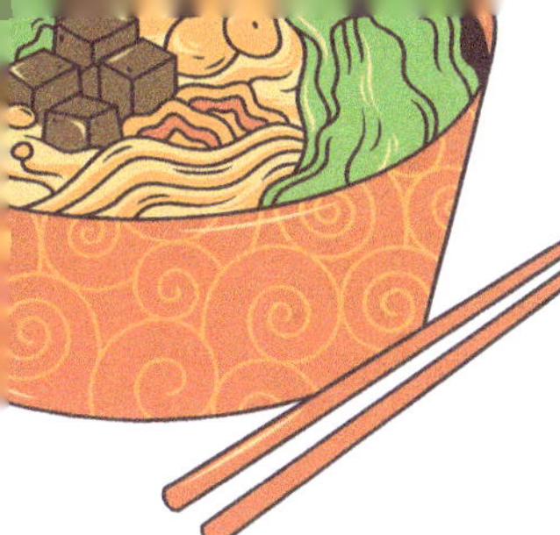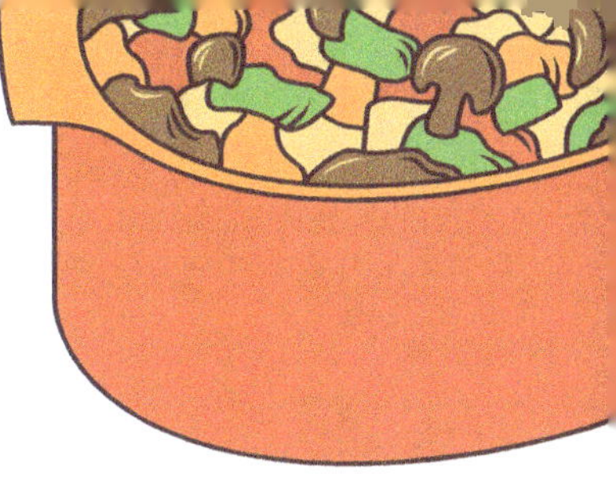

COMMON COOKING MEASUREMENTS

Weight Measurements

MEASUREMENT	EQUIVALENT
1 ounce (oz)	28.35 grams (g)
1 pound (lb)	16 ounces (oz)
1 kilogram (kg)	2.2 pounds (lbs)

Liquid Measurements

MEASUREMENT	EQUIVALENT
1 fluid ounce (fl oz)	2 tablespoons (tbsp)
1 cup	8 fluid ounces (fl oz)
1 pint (pt)	16 fluid ounces (fl oz)
1 quart (qt)	32 fluid ounces (fl oz)
1 gallon (gal)	128 fluid ounces (fl oz)

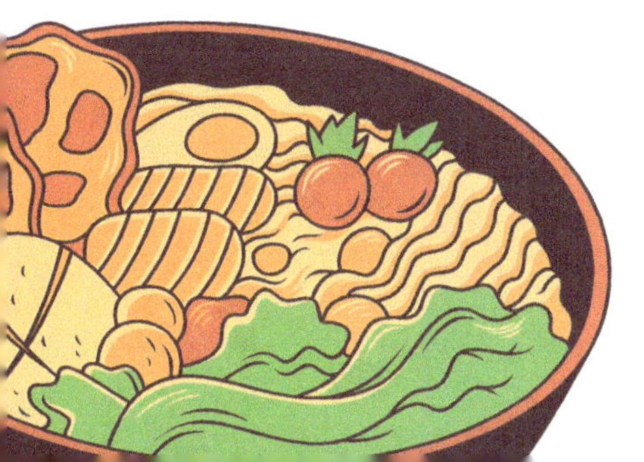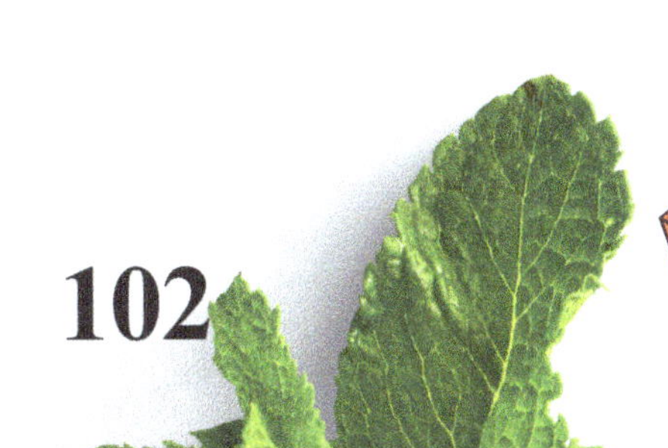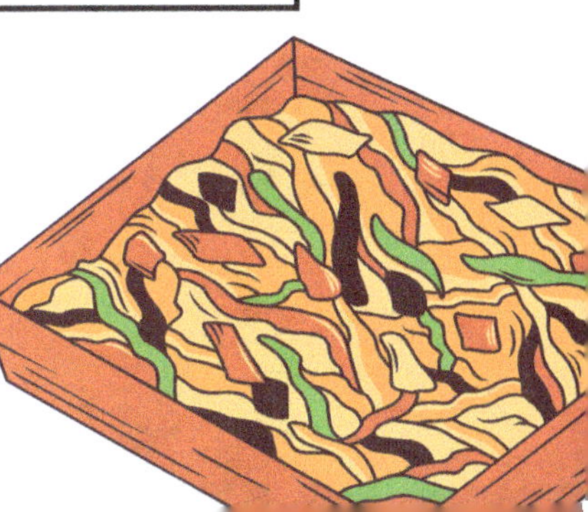

OVEN TEMPERATURES
Temperature Conversions

FAHRENHEIT (°F)	CELSIUS (°C)	GAS MARK
250°F	120°C	1/2
275°F	135°C	1
300°F	150°C	2
325°F	165°C	3
350°F	175°C	4
375°F	190°C	5
400°F	200°C	6
425°F	220°C	7
450°F	230°C	8
475°F	245°C	9
500°F	260°C	10

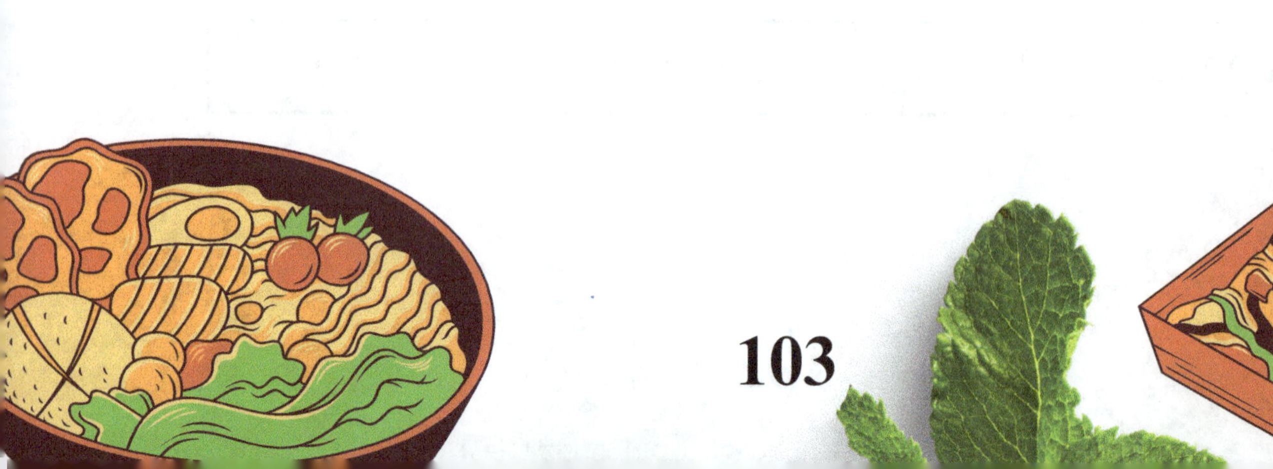

METRIC CONVERSIONS

Volume

METRIC	U.S. EQUIVALENT
1 milliliter (ml)	0.034 fluid ounces (fl oz)
100 milliliters	3.4 fluid ounces (fl oz)
1 liter (l)	34 fluid ounces (fl oz)
1 liter (l)	4.2 cups
1 liter (l)	2.1 pints

Weight

METRIC	U.S. EQUIVALENT
1 gram (g)	0.035 ounces (oz)
100 grams (g)	3.5 ounces (oz)
500 grams (g)	17.6 ounces (oz)
1 kilogram (kg)	2.2 pounds (lbs)

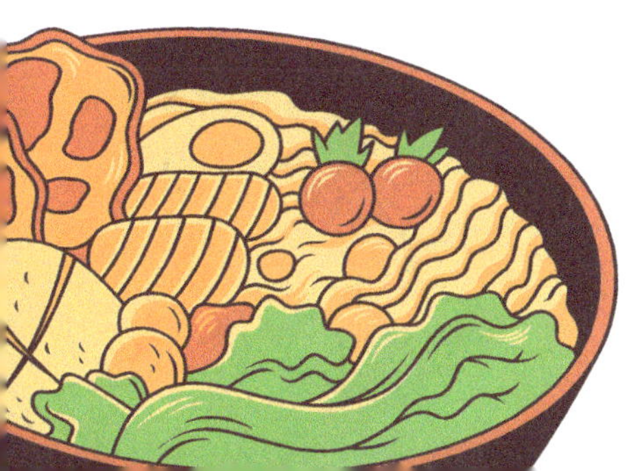
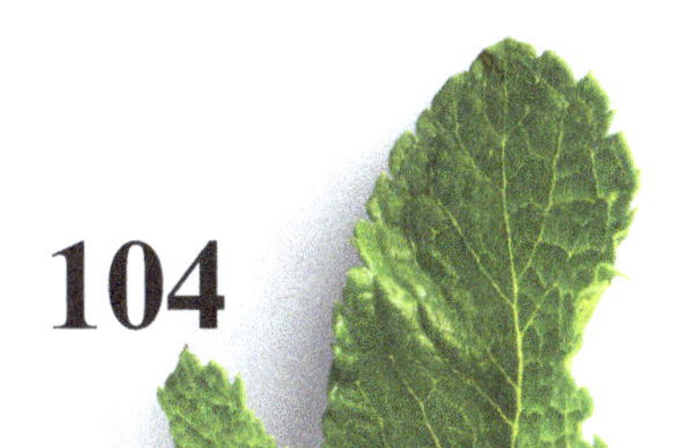
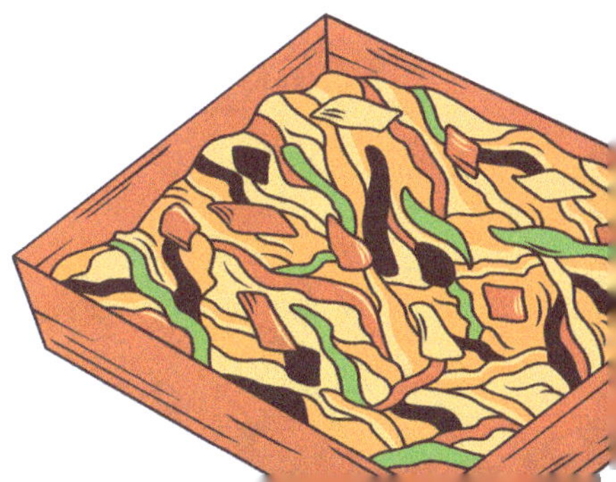

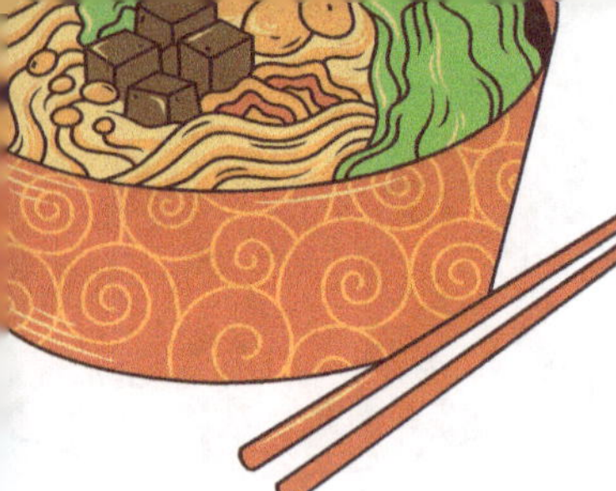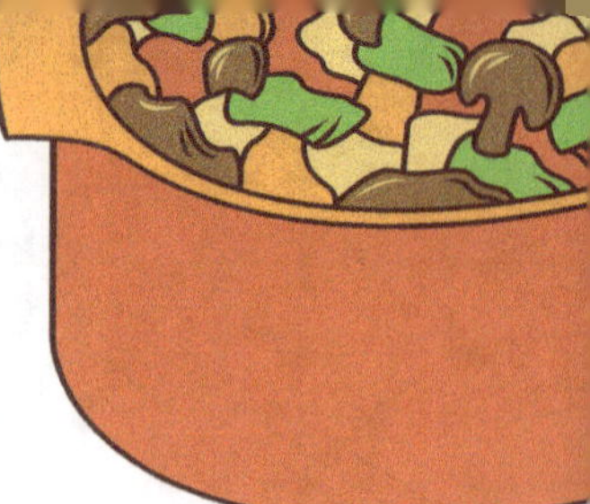

COMMON COOKING MEASUREMENTS

Volume Measurements

MEASUREMENT	EQUIVALENT
tsp	teaspoon
tbsp	tablespoon
Cup	Cup
oz	ounce
lb	pound
ml	milliliter
l	liter
g	gram
Kg	Kilogram
fl oz	fluid ounce

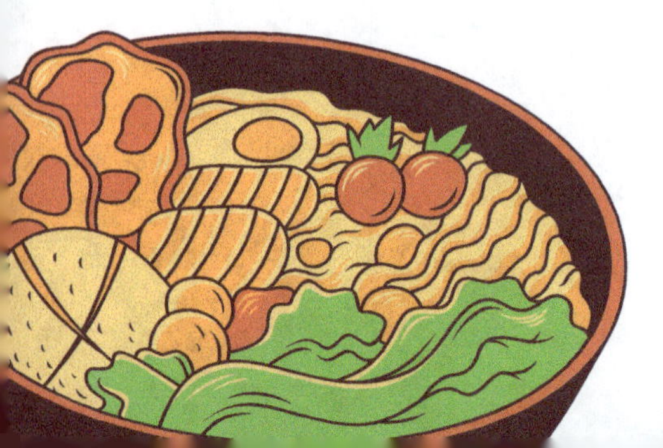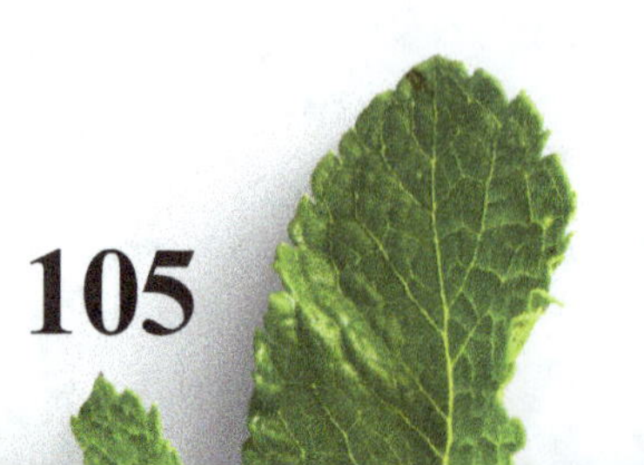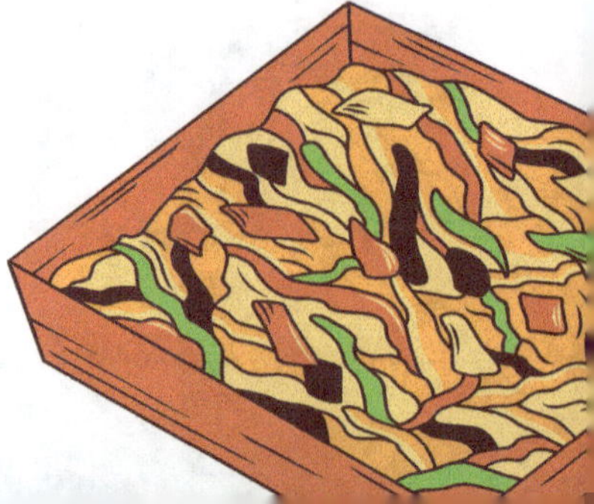

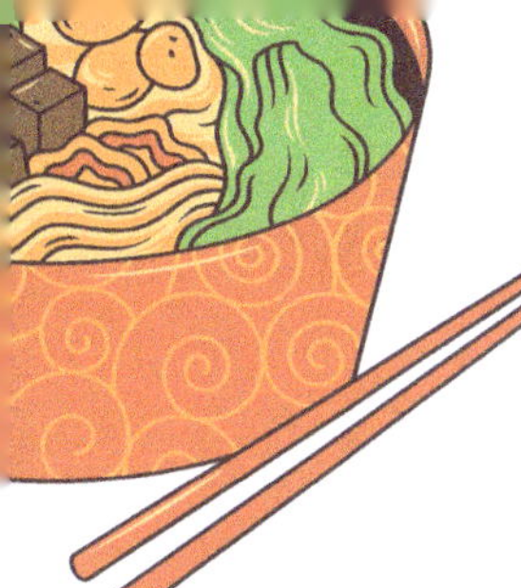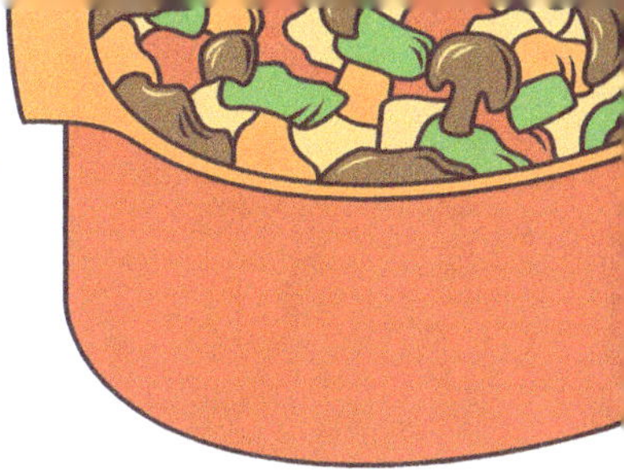

COMMON COOKING MEASUREMENTS

Volume Measurements

1 cup all-purpose flour = 120 grams
1 cup granulated sugar = 200 grams
1 cup brown sugar = 220 grams
1 cup butter = 227 grams (or 2 sticks)
1 large egg = 50 grams

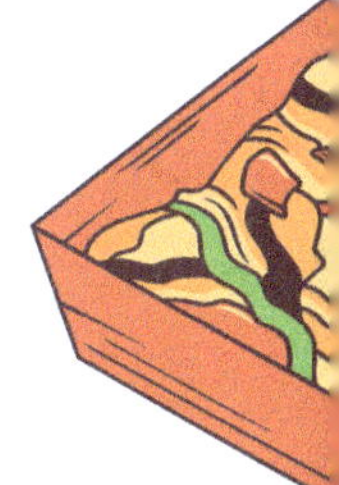

Note:

- When measuring dry ingredients, use a spoon to fill the measuring cup or spoon, and level off with a flat edge for accuracy.
- For liquid ingredients, use a clear measuring cup and check at eye level.
- When converting recipes, be mindful of the precision required for baking versus cooking.

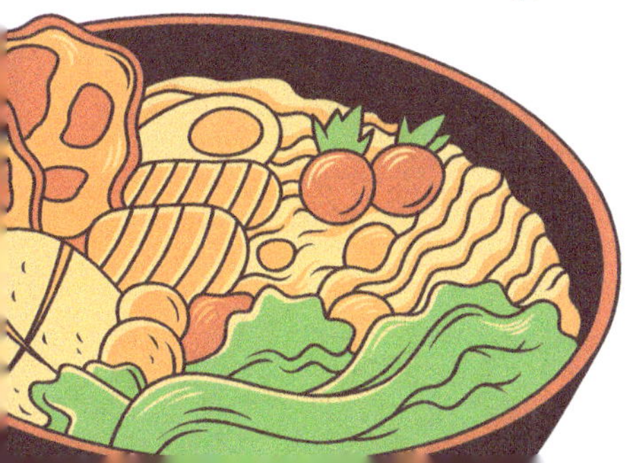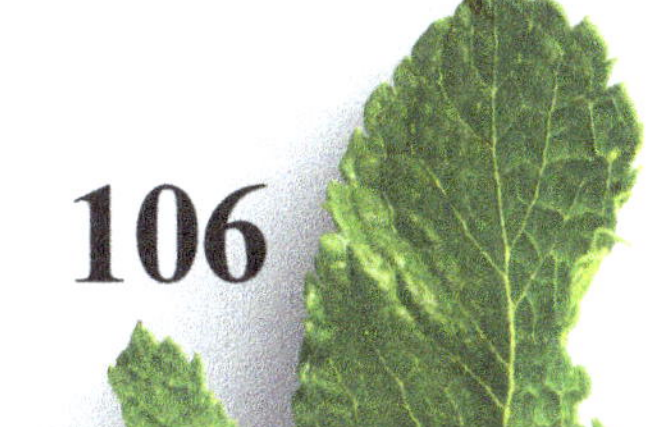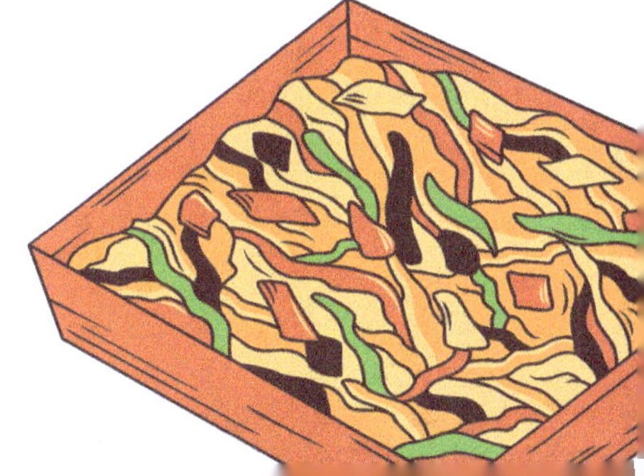

GLOSSARY

General Nutrition Terms

1. **Anti-Inflammatory Foods**: Foods that help reduce inflammation, such as leafy greens, fatty fish, nuts, and berries.

2. **Nutrient-Dense**: Foods that are high in essential nutrients like vitamins, minerals, and antioxidants relative to their calorie content.

3. **Gluten-Free**: Foods that do not contain gluten, a protein found in wheat, barley, and rye, often used for those with gluten sensitivities or celiac disease.

4. **Dairy-Free**: Foods that do not contain milk or milk products, are suitable for those who are lactose intolerant or allergic to dairy.

5. **Omega-3 Fatty Acids**: Essential fats found in foods like fish, flaxseeds, and walnuts that have anti-inflammatory properties and support heart health.

6. **Antioxidants:** Compounds found in foods like fruits and vegetables that protect cells from damage caused by free radicals.

7. **Whole Grains:** Grains that contain all parts of the grain kernel, such as brown rice, quinoa, and oats, provide more nutrients and fibre compared to refined grains.

8. **Legumes:** A group of plant foods that include beans, lentils, peas, and chickpeas, known for being high in protein, fibre, and other nutrients.

9. **Leafy Greens:** Vegetables like spinach, kale, and arugula that are high in vitamins, minerals, and antioxidants.

10. **Fermented Foods**: Foods that have been through a fermentation process, such as yoghurt, kimchi, and sauerkraut, contain beneficial probiotics.

11. **Probiotics:** Beneficial bacteria in fermented foods support gut health and the immune system.

12. **Gluten**: A protein in wheat, barley, and rye that some people need to avoid due to celiac disease or gluten sensitivity.

General Nutrition Terms

13. **Lactose**: A sugar found in milk and dairy products that some people cannot digest properly, leading to lactose intolerance.

14. **Phytochemicals**: Compounds produced by plants that have health benefits, such as flavonoids and carotenoids, found in colourful fruits and vegetables.

15. **Superfoods**: Nutrient-rich foods considered to be especially beneficial for health and well-being, like blueberries, salmon, and spinach.

16. **Healthy Fats:** Fats that are beneficial for health, such as monounsaturated and polyunsaturated fats found in foods like avocados, nuts, and olive oil.

17. **Refined Sugars:** Sugars that have been processed and stripped of nutrients, such as white sugar and high-fructose corn syrup, which can contribute to inflammation.

18. **Phytonutrients**: Natural compounds found in plants that have various health benefits, including antioxidant and anti-inflammatory effects.

19. **Low-Glycemic Foods:** Foods that have a low impact on blood sugar levels, such as most vegetables, some fruits, and whole grains.

20. **Detoxification**: The process of removing toxins from the body, often through diet and hydration.

21. **Micronutrients**: Essential vitamins and minerals are needed in small amounts for proper body function.

22. **Macros**: Short for macronutrients, which include carbohydrates, proteins, and fats, the main components of our diet.

23. **Plant-Based:** Diets that primarily consist of plant foods like vegetables, fruits, grains, nuts, and seeds, with minimal or no animal products.

24. **Saturated Fats:** Fats are typically found in animal products and some plant oils that should be consumed in moderation.

General Nutrition Terms

25. **Unsaturated Fats:** Healthy fats found in plants and fish, beneficial for heart health and overall wellness.

26. **Whole Foods**: Foods that are minimally processed and closer to their natural form, such as fresh fruits and vegetables, whole grains, and lean proteins.

27. **Meal Prep**: The process of preparing meals in advance to save time and ensure healthy eating throughout the week.

28. **Hydration**: Maintaining an adequate level of fluid in the body to support all bodily functions, often emphasized in healthy eating plans.

29. **Flaxseeds:** Small seeds high in omega-3 fatty acids, fiber, and antioxidants, often used to boost nutrition in meals.

30. **Chia Seeds:** Tiny seeds rich in omega-3 fatty acids, fiber, and protein, commonly added to smoothies and cereals for added nutrition.

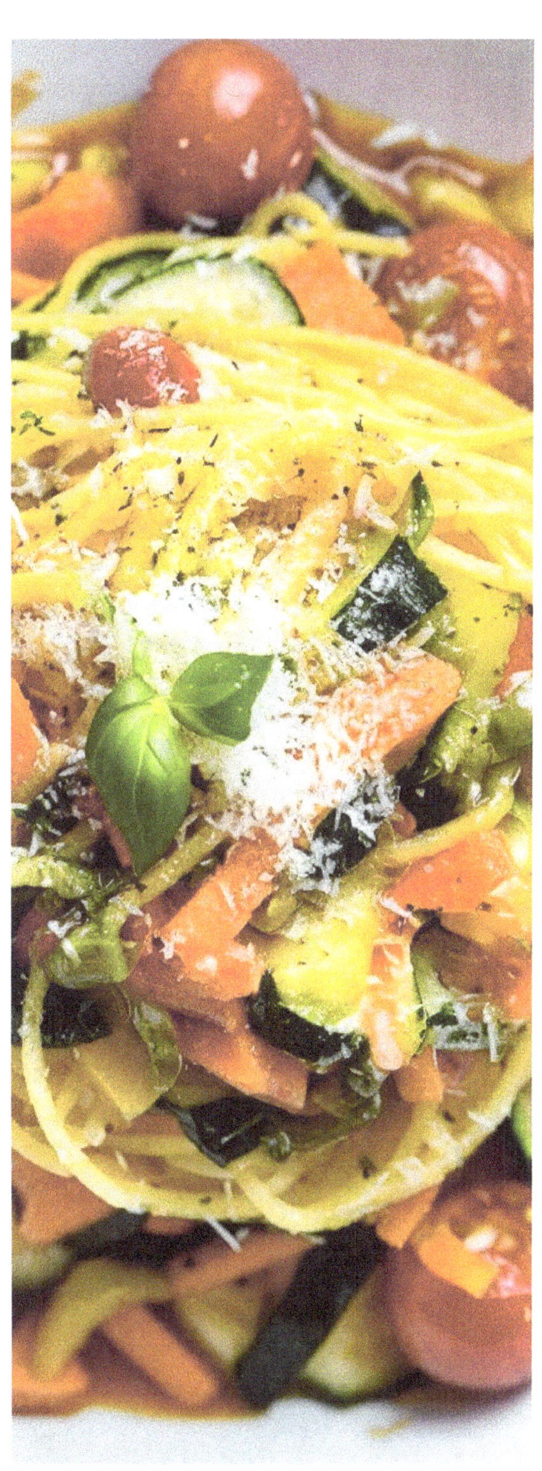

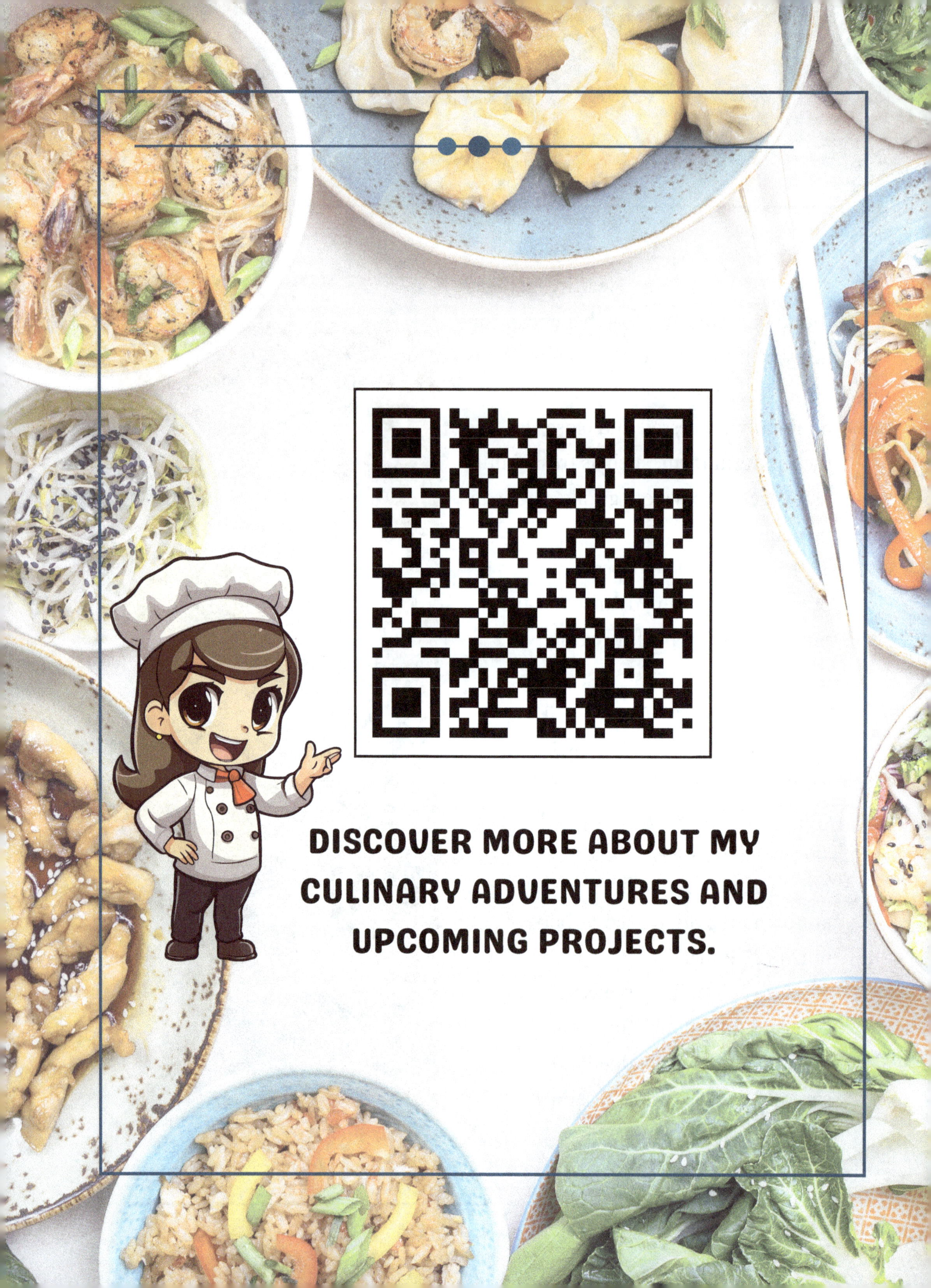
DISCOVER MORE ABOUT MY
CULINARY ADVENTURES AND
UPCOMING PROJECTS.

THE AUTHOR

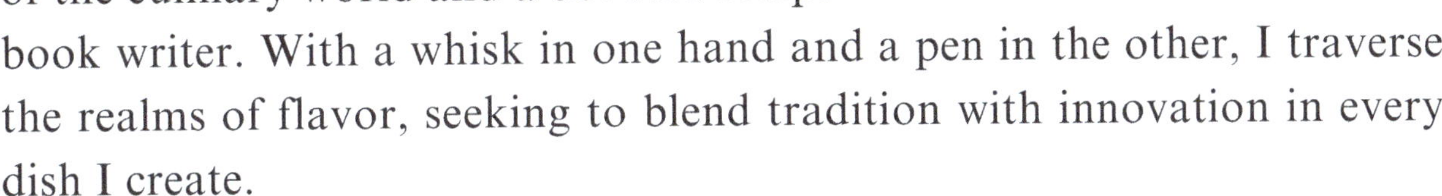

Hello, culinary adventurers!
I'm Vakare Rimkute, a passionate explorer of the culinary world and a devoted recipe book writer. With a whisk in one hand and a pen in the other, I traverse the realms of flavor, seeking to blend tradition with innovation in every dish I create.

Growing up in the bustling kitchens of my Lithuanian grandmother, I developed an insatiable curiosity for the alchemy of ingredients and the magic they could weave on the palate. From the rustic charm of hearty stews to the delicate intricacies of pastries, my journey through food has been nothing short of a delightful adventure.

After years of experimenting and honing my craft, I found my true calling as a recipe book writer. With each recipe I pen, I aim to capture the essence of culinary culture while infusing it with a touch of modern flair. From comforting classics to bold culinary experiments, my recipes are a reflection of my belief that food should not only nourish the body but also nourish the soul.

So join me on this gastronomic journey, where every page is filled with tantalizing flavors, heartwarming stories, and a dash of humor. Together, let's embark on a culinary adventure that will tickle your taste buds and leave you craving for more. Happy cooking!